Table of Contents

Golden Cure

The Alchemy of Healing with Gold and Selenium

by

Dr. ant

No part of this book may be reproduced in any form or by any electronic or mechanical means including information storage and retrieval systems, without permission in writing from the author. The only exception is by a reviewer, who may quote short excerpts in a review.

Although the author and publisher have made every effort to ensure that the information in this book was correct at press time, the author and publisher do not assume and hereby disclaim any liability to any party for any loss, damage, or disruption caused by errors or omissions, whether such errors or omissions result from negligence, accident, or any other cause.

This publication is designed to provide accurate and authoritative information with regard to the subject matter covered. It is sold with the understanding that the publisher is not engaged in rendering professional services. If legal advice or other expert assistance is required, the services of a competent professional should be sought.

The fact that an organization or website is referred to in this work as a citation and/or a potential source of further information does not mean that the author or the publisher endorses the information the organization or website may provide or recommendations it may make.

Please remember that Internet websites listed in this work may have changed or disappeared between when this work was written and when it is read.

Golden Cure: The Alchemy of Healing with Gold and Selenium

Contents

Introduction

In a world where science often dances on the edge of the known and the unknown, there's a growing curiosity about the hidden potentials of substances like gold and selenium. While these elements have been engaged in a scientific tug-of-war between skepticism and admiration, they continue to intrigue health-conscious individuals and medical professionals alike. This book ventures into that liminal space where ancient wisdom meets modern research, aiming to illuminate the untapped possibilities and engage you in meaningful discourse.

Our journey begins by probing the mysterious allure of monoatomic gold, a subject whose complexities have fueled myriad theories. Scholars and enthusiasts have long debated its properties. Is it a mystical cure-all or grounded in biochemical reality? We'll explore the historical roots of gold in medicine, revealing rituals and remedies from civilizations that saw within this metal something far more precious than its sheen. We aim to uncover how perceptions have evolved over centuries, leading up to today's scientific inquiries and societal beliefs.

No investigation of monoatomic gold would be complete without a parallel examination of selenium, an element whose reputation oscillates between essential nutrient and miracle cure. While renowned for its role in human health, selenium also represents a puzzle within medical science. How does it fit within the spectrum of alternative and traditional medicine? We'll sketch a portrait of its evolving place in modern healthcare systems, and question whether it's more than just another player in the nutritional orchestra.

The intersection of alchemy and science is one of the most intriguing convergences addressed in our exploration. Alchemy, once dismissed as mumbo jumbo, increasingly finds its echoes in modern scientific practices. We'll delve into how ancient practices of alchemy have influenced, and been legitimized by, contemporary scientific validations. It's a compelling narrative where age-old methodologies are reinterpreted through the lens of modern analytical tools, inviting not just acceptance, but respect.

The intrigue doesn't stop at theoretical discussions. Gold's potential as a cancer treatment is being scrutinized in clinical studies and evaluated through patient anecdotes, highlighting a deeply human aspect of scientific inquiry. How can personal experiences inform broader medical practices? And where do anecdotal claims stand in a world that prioritizes empirical evidence? We'll think deeply about how individual stories add layers of complexity to the scientific landscape, challenging traditional methods of assessment.

Complementing this is selenium's role in cancer prevention. Analyzed through the rigors of scientific inquiry and real-world applications, the narrative around selenium shifts from speculation to potentially groundbreaking insight. By examining case studies, we illuminate its place on the fine line between inspiration and evidence, reinforcing our central theme: health substances often live in a liminal space, straddling the sacred and the scientific.

The combined effects of gold and selenium present opportunities for further inquiry into collective potentials. This dual engagement not only raises questions about biochemical interactions but suggests a synergy that may reframe our understanding of these elements in medical contexts. Though sometimes met with skepticism, the idea of combined treatments provides fertile ground for challenging and paradigmatic shifts in healthcare perspectives.

Yet, it's critical to address the controversy that shadows alternative treatments. From an investigative angle, we'll dissect skepticism and engage with criticisms of these therapies, weighing their merits and limitations. In navigating these contentious waters, we're tasked with balancing criticism with consideration, facts with possibilities, always with the end goal of transparency and informed understanding.

The methodologies underpinning scientific research will also be a topic of discussion. How do we measure the efficacy of treatments that lie at the fringes of traditional practice? The integrity of a study, its peer reviews, and the empirical methodologies employed all form the backbone of our analysis. Our aim is to embolden the reader with tools to critically assess alternative therapies alongside mainstream options.

In an era of increasing dialogue around alternative medicine, the ethical dimensions of treatment choices cannot be ignored. We'll probe the delicate balance between scientific rigor and the often desperate hope for healing. What ethical dilemmas arise when science and subjective experience intersect? These musings foster a broader conversation about what it means to ethically engage with treatment options that lie outside the norm.

Legal frameworks provide yet another layer of complexity. As alternative medicine gains prominence, regulatory landscapes struggle to keep pace. Exploring challenges and precedents offers insight into the legal environment that influences both practitioners and patients. Our intention is to demystify these regulations to provide a clearer pathway for those navigating the complexities of alternative medicine.

Throughout the narrative, case studies of recovery provide real-world validation, anchoring the theoretical with personal triumphs. These stories bring human faces to facts, adding depth to numbers and statistics, and affirming the potential for transformation. By giving voice to those who have walked the path of alternative treatments, we can glean lessons that inspire and educate.

Yet, no investigation would be complete without acknowledging the risks and side effects associated with alternative treatments. Our exploration aims to identify potential adverse reactions and strategies to manage associated risks. Informed choices require a broad perspective, encompassing both promises and pitfalls.

As the narrative unfolds, we'll delve into the integration of traditional and alternative medicine. It's a complex dance between worlds, requiring understanding from both scientific practitioners and holistic health advocates. By seeking common ground, we pave the way for more comprehensive approaches to health and healing.

Nutritional dimensions also take center stage, with diet and supplementation forming the bedrock of both traditional and alternative health strategies. What roles do gold and selenium play in these approaches? From nutritional strategies to mental and emotional dimensions of healing, we'll explore holistic perspectives that honor the body and mind connection.

Ultimately, this book aims to be more than just a repository of knowledge. It's an invitation to question, reflect, and engage with the evolving landscape of health and medicine. As we explore the intricacies of gold and selenium, our goal is to foster a deeper understanding, one that truly bridges the old with the new, the mystical with the empirical.

Chapter 1: The Mystique of Monoatomic Gold

Monoatomic gold, a subject of both fascination and skepticism in the realm of alternative medicine, beckons curiosity with its purported ability to heal and transform. It's a substance that, despite its unassuming appearance, has captivated the imagination and sparked debates on its mysterious effects on health. Those who advocate for its use suggest that monoatomic gold might influence brain function, enhance spiritual well-being, and even bolster physical health. Yet, the scientific community remains divided. Historical narratives hint at gold's revered status as a medicinal element across cultures, whispering promises of rejuvenation and vitality. Whether these anecdotes possess merit or are mere echoes of ancient alchemy, they invite a deeper investigation. Understanding monoatomic gold requires an exploration that balances anecdotal claims with rigorous scientific inquiry, challenging us to look beyond traditional paradigms and contemplate the possibilities this element might hold in today's search for holistic healing.

Understanding Monoatomic Elements

The enigmatic allure of monoatomic elements lies in their unique atomic structure, which diverges dramatically from the conventional elements familiar to us. At its core, a monoatomic element exists in a single atomic state, harmoniously isolated without forming bonds with other atoms. This distinctiveness bestows upon it a range of properties that have intrigued scientists, alchemists, and alternative medicine enthusiasts alike.

To delve deeper into the science, an element typically bonds with similar atoms to create the molecules and compounds constituting our tangible world. Yet, monoatomic elements defy this principle. In a monoatomic state, elements such as gold, platinum, and iridium exist independently, devoid of the molecular chains and lattices that define their conventional guise. This labile state has generated discussions around their energetic qualities and potential health impacts.

As we pivot from the structure to the purported properties, discussions often arise around their energy and vibrational frequency. Some proponents assert that these elements possess enhanced bioavailability, enabling the body to harness their benefits more effectively. The debate continues regarding how these particles interact at a cellular level and whether they can truly influence physiological processes, resulting in health benefits touted by alternative medicine practitioners.

Among the most captivating narratives accompanying monoatomic elements is their storied past. Ancient alchemists like those of Egypt and China were captivated by the pursuit of transforming base metals into noble ones, often focusing on gold. Although modern science discerns no material transmutation, the fascination with monoatomic states—their potential to mimic the transformative power of alchemy—remains potent. This historical allure contributes to the mystique, infusing the subject with a blend of reverence and skepticism.

In the realm of health and wellness, monoatomic elements draw both intrigue and controversy. Advocates suggest these elements, when ingested or applied, foster increased mental clarity, bolster vitality, and even enhance spiritual awareness. However, their use is not without controversy. Critics argue a scarcity of rigorous scientific backing to substantiate such claims, urging caution and further investigation. The field teeters on the edge of anecdotal enthusiasm and scientific ambiguity, demanding a thorough examination of available evidence.

Navigating the scientific landscape of monoatomic elements requires discernment, particularly due to the complex interplay between quantum physics and chemistry. At this confluence, researchers explore potential shifts in physical properties at a nano-scale—transformations that might bestow monoatomic elements with attributes unknown to their bulk counterparts. The notion that structure at the atomic level can impact elemental behavior fuels ongoing inquiry and curiosity.

One can't ignore the advent of modern technology in shaping our understanding of these elusive elements. Advances in spectroscopy and electron microscopy provide unprecedented insights, allowing researchers to visualize and manipulate atoms with surgical precision. These tools empower scientists to corroborate characteristics once relegated to the realm of speculative alchemy, bridging the gap between age-old legends and tangible evidence.

Moreover, as we venture into the chemical potential of monoatomic elements, it's crucial to consider their role as catalysts. Their unique atomic spacing and surface area can influence reactions in unexpected ways. This potential has implications not just in theoretical chemistry but also in practical applications, from pharmaceuticals to industrial processes, hinting at a utility that transcends mere therapeutic use.

The investigation into monoatomic elements intersects with broader themes of essential nutrients and alternative treatment modalities. While the focus often zeroes in on monoatomic gold due to its historical prominence and high regard, monoatomic forms of other elements also warrant exploration in their respective capacities. Each element, with its distinctive properties, might offer different therapeutic or practical advantages, meriting individual study and contemplation.

Understanding monoatomic elements is not merely an intellectual endeavor but also a multifaceted journey through the intersections of culture, science, and medicine. Whether they're seen as harbingers of a new therapeutic paradigm or remnants of hallowed alchemical tradition, they challenge us to rethink our preconceptions of elemental nature. This odyssey may yet unveil new facets of the chemical universe, transforming age-old mysteries into concrete knowledge. As we proceed, the balance between optimism and skepticism will undoubtedly guide the path of discovery.

Historical Perspectives on Gold as Medicine

Gold, with its lustrous allure, has long fascinated humans, not just for its economic value but also for its purported therapeutic properties. Throughout history, civilizations have turned to this precious metal, exploring its potential as a medicinal substance. While modern science approaches with skepticism, the ancients were curious and bold, often attributing magical attributes to gold's enigmatic nature.

In ancient Egypt, gold's mystique was fortified by its association with deities and immortality. The Egyptians believed gold to be indestructible and divine, often crafting it into amulets and ornaments buried with pharaohs. But beyond adornment, gold was also ingested. The Egyptians may have believed in its capacity to rejuvenate, using gold dust mixed with other substances to maintain health and stave off disease. This use was perhaps as much symbolic as it was based on observed benefits, but it laid the groundwork for gold's journey into medicinal lore.

Moving east to ancient China, gold was equally revered. The Taoists, pioneers in proto-chemistry and alchemy, sought the "elixir of life," a legendary potion granting immortality. Gold featured prominently in their experiments, often consumed in the hope of achieving longevity and spiritual enlightenment. In traditional Chinese medicine, gold was thought to balance elemental forces within the body, contributing to the overall harmony essential for good health.

The Greeks and Romans, influenced by their predecessors, also explored gold's potential. They utilized it for various ailments, including mental health issues. Pliny the Elder documented gold's use as a remedy for wounds and mental disturbances, demonstrating an early understanding of the potential psychological benefits of gold. While empirical evidence was lacking, gold's use was justified by its rarity and inherent value.

In medieval Europe, alchemy reached its zenith, intertwining mystical beliefs with nascent scientific inquiry. Alchemists sought not only to transmute base metals into gold but to harness its perceived medicinal properties. "Aurum potabile" or "drinkable gold," was a concoction believed to cure ailments and extend life. However, the practice remained shrouded in secrecy, often dismissed by later generations as pseudoscience.

As the Enlightenment dawned, bringing a new age of reason, the medicinal use of gold did not entirely fade. The 19th century saw a more scientific approach. Gold was explored as a treatment for conditions like rheumatoid arthritis, with patients receiving gold injections in hopes of reducing inflammation. This marked a shift from alchemic traditions to attempts at evidence-based medicine, setting the stage for ongoing research into gold's therapeutic properties.

Despite its ancient roots, gold as medicine was not without controversy. As with many alternative treatments, skepticism has shadowed its history. Yet, this skepticism could not completely extinguish interest. Cultures worldwide maintained a fascination with gold, rooted in its alleged ability to heal and maintain youth. Though scientifically unsubstantiated for much of its history, gold lingered as a symbol of hope.

From the Egyptians to the Taoists, the use of gold in medicine underscores a universal yearning for health and longevity. Cultures separated by geography and time converged in their reverence for this metal, driven by a common quest for wellness and balance. The historical narratives of gold in medicine are layered with intrigue and reflect an enduring human curiosity about the natural world.

Today, the legacy of gold in medicine is being reassessed under the microscope of modern science. Research seeks to isolate the potential health benefits tied to gold compounds, delving deeper than records of antiquity could. Despite varied historical applications and beliefs that sometimes bordered on myth, gold remains a subject of fascination in the context of medicinal use. Its allure persists, challenging us to discern fact from fiction in the search for healing.

Chapter 2: The Role of Selenium in Health

Selenium, an essential trace mineral, finds itself at the intersection of health and controversy. It's both a critical nutrient and a subject of modern medical intrigue, revealing layers of potential roles that extend beyond basic nutrition. In a balanced diet, selenium supports the immune system, enhances cognitive function, and plays a vital role in thyroid health. Its antioxidant properties help mitigate oxidative stress, reducing the risk of chronic diseases. Medical professionals continue to explore selenium's breadth of influence, as studies evaluate its complex biological mechanisms and therapeutic possibilities. Described sometimes as a miracle cure, the nuanced reality calls for careful consideration and ongoing research. Understanding selenium's role helps frame its impact on overall well-being, offering a compelling look at what might be a small, yet mighty player in the grand scheme of health. This chapter interrogates these aspects, inviting readers to ponder selenium's full potential in our journey towards health optimization.

Essential Nutrient or Miracle Cure?

Selenium, a trace mineral that plays a pivotal role in many metabolic pathways, has piqued the interest of both nutritionists and proponents of alternative medicine. Its dual identity as an essential nutrient and a potential miracle cure adds layers of complexity that deserve exploration. As we delve into the nuances of selenium's role in health, the question arises: is it simply an indispensable component of our diet, or does it hold the promise of transformative healing?

The intrigue surrounding selenium often begins with its necessity for human health. This mineral contributes to numerous physiological functions, most notably its role as a key player in antioxidant defense. Part of glutathione peroxidase, a crucial enzyme, selenium helps protect cells from oxidative damage and supports a robust immune system. Its influence extends to thyroid hormone metabolism and even the synthesis of DNA. In these capacities, selenium is undeniably essential. A deficiency can lead to a host of problems, including Keshan disease, a potentially fatal heart disorder, and Kashin-Beck disease, a chronic bone condition.

Yet, it is selenium's potential beyond basic nutrition that fuels ongoing interest. Its purported capabilities as a miracle cure provoke both fascination and skepticism. Initial evidence suggested a possible link between selenium supplementation and cancer prevention. Observational studies hinted that higher selenium intake might correlate with a decreased risk of certain cancers, propelling further research into its prophylactic possibilities. However, subsequent results have been mixed, leaving the scientific community and public alike in limbo about selenium's efficacy as a cancer-fighting agent.

In considering selenium's dual roles, it's crucial to examine the fine line between therapeutic benefits and toxicity. Selenium's biological activity is both powerful and, when taken in excessive amounts, potentially harmful. This narrow therapeutic window underscores the importance of caution in supplementation. Furthermore, with regional soil depletions and dietary variations affecting selenium intake, achieving optimal balance can be tricky. Consuming the mineral within recommended limits is imperative to harness its health benefits without inviting adverse effects.

Nonetheless, the narrative of selenium as a miraculous agent isn't solely anchored in cancer prevention. Its speculated neurological benefits have attracted attention, too. Some studies suggest that selenium may play a role in neuroprotection, potentially mitigating conditions like Alzheimer's disease. As oxidative stress becomes increasingly linked to neurodegenerative disorders, the enzyme-dependent antioxidant properties of selenium come into sharper focus. While findings offer glimmers of hope, rigorous scientific scrutiny and validation are required to substantiate these claims.

A significant factor propelling selenium's status in alternative medicine is anecdotal evidence. Testimonials often circulate about its impact on vitality, immune resilience, and overall well-being. Such accounts, while compelling, must be approached with discernment, understanding the difference between isolated personal experiences and generalizable scientific findings. The allure of selenium as a cure-all solution may hinge on persuasive stories, but these narratives need support from systematic research.

Undoubtedly, selenium's reputation as an essential nutrient is well-earned. Its undeniable role in maintaining vital bodily functions solidifies its importance in our diet. However, when we transition from acknowledging its necessity to exploring its potential as a versatile therapeutic agent, the conversation becomes more complex. Scientific investigation, while promising in some respects, has yet to conclusively validate selenium as a stand-alone miracle cure. The task of unraveling selenium's mechanisms calls for careful, methodical study backed by robust clinical trials.

The allure of miracle cures is a recurrent theme in the search for holistic wellbeing, and selenium encapsulates this quest. It's a journey that must balance curiosity with caution. While pursuing new horizons in health sciences is vital, the responsibility to ground such explorations in scientific reality remains paramount.

Ultimately, whether selenium stands as a quintessential nutrient or an emblem of miraculous healing hinges on ongoing research. As new studies continue to probe its potential, illuminating the path forward, what remains clear is the multifaceted nature of this fascinating element. For now, selenium's story is one of potential, of a substance with known foundational roles and tantalizing promise, requiring further exploration to unearth its full implications in human health.

Selenium in Modern Medicine

In the ever-evolving landscape of modern medicine, selenium has found its place as more than just a trace element necessary for human health. It stands at the intersection of traditional nutrition and cutting-edge medical science, provoking intrigue among health professionals and researchers alike. From its essential role in metabolism to its unexpected potential in cancer therapies, selenium navigates multiple fronts in medical research.

Selenium's contribution to human health, especially its powerful antioxidant properties, cannot be overstated. Its ability to combat oxidative stress—a known factor in numerous diseases—has positioned it as a potential agent in the prevention of various chronic conditions. Selenium contributes to the activity of enzymes like glutathione peroxidases and thioredoxin reductases, which are keys to cellular defense mechanisms in combating oxidative damage. This biochemical relationship has spurred further investigations into how selenium supplementation could prove beneficial in clinical settings.

In the realm of endocrinology, selenium's influence on thyroid function is particularly noteworthy. The element is critical for the conversion of thyroid hormones, which regulate metabolism and impact nearly every cell in the body. Clinical observations indicate that selenium supplementation might assist in managing autoimmune thyroid conditions like Hashimoto's thyroiditis. These insights have directed some endocrinologists to explore selenium as part of integrative treatment plans for thyroid disorders. While the results are promising, the medical community remains cautious until comprehensive clinical trials deliver conclusive evidence.

The intersection of selenium with oncology is an area rife with both excitement and skepticism. Studies suggest selenium's potential in reducing the risk of certain types of cancer, including prostate, colorectal, and lung cancers. Researchers are delving into the ways selenium may influence carcinogenic processes, with hypotheses centered around apoptosis induction and DNA repair enhancement. These anti-carcinogenic properties make selenium a candidate for chemoprevention strategies. However, despite a flurry of encouraging data, the scientific community remains divided, with some studies showing no substantial benefits in selenium supplementation for cancer prevention.

In cardiovascular health, selenium seems to exert a protective effect through its inclusion in selenoproteins that aid in reducing inflammation and improving vascular health. Epidemiological studies have reported lower selenium levels associated with increased risk of cardiovascular diseases. While the benefits of selenium in cardiovascular medicine are persuasive, the outcomes of research are not uniformly consistent. The nuanced relationship between selenium levels, genetic factors, and disease outcomes continues to be an important area of study, potentially unlocking more sophisticated approaches to cardiovascular therapy.

The application of selenium in infectious disease management is another evolving frontier. Its ability to support immune system function could make it an adjunct in managing viral infections. For instance, research into selenium's role in HIV management points to improved immune function and reduced disease progression in selenium-supplemented individuals. Although far from being a standalone treatment, these findings illustrate selenium's potential in complementing existing treatment regimens.

Moreover, selenium's burgeoning role in integrative medicine provides a backdrop for exploring its synergy with other mineral and vitamin supplements. Its interaction with elements like vitamin E has revealed potential in enhancing antioxidant defenses. This synergy is also apparent in settings where selenium is combined with conventional treatments, potentially reducing side effects and improving patient outcomes. Yet, despite these potential benefits, caution is advised due to the narrow therapeutic index of selenium, where both deficiency and excess pose health risks.

The technological innovations in medical research also bolster the understanding of selenium's place in healthcare. Advanced bioinformatics and medical imaging techniques have allowed for precise observations of selenium's effects at the molecular level. Computational models are increasingly used to predict selenium's interactions within biological systems, providing novel insights and refining therapeutic interventions. These advancements position selenium as a pivotal subject in the broader narrative of personalized medicine, where customized approaches consider an individual's unique biochemical makeup.

Despite these advances, the incorporation of selenium into mainstream medical practice faces hurdles. Regulatory pathways complicate the approval process for selenium-based therapies, given the existing divide in clinical findings. Moreover, the ethical concerns of promoting selenium in clinical practice without unequivocal evidence demand balanced discourse and thorough peer review. Medical professionals are thus urged to remain informed, weighing current evidence against evolving research to responsibly guide treatment decisions.

Ultimately, the narrative of selenium in modern medicine is one of possibility tempered by caution. It is a story characterized by potent potential that challenges traditional boundaries, urging a reevaluation of what is deemed possible within the confines of modern pharmacology. As continued research peels back layers of the selenium enigma, the medical community may indeed find that this trace element holds keys to unlocking new therapeutic frontiers that have yet to be fully explored.

Chapter 3: Alchemy Rediscovered

The ancient art of alchemy, long dismissed as the stuff of fantasy and superstition, is experiencing a resurgence in the realm of modern science and medicine. Unlike medieval alchemists intent on transmuting lead into gold, today's explorers are uncovering how alchemical principles might inform novel approaches to healing. By reevaluating ancient practices through the lens of contemporary scientific inquiry, we gain insights into how these age-old methods could bridge the gap between mystical traditions and empirical research. Strands of historical wisdom intertwine with cutting-edge discoveries, urging both health-conscious individuals and medical professionals to consider alchemical practices in a new light. The fusion of ancient and modern ideas underscores a renewed curiosity about whether these practices offer tangible benefits, sparking a dialogue that challenges our understanding of health and healing.

Ancient Alchemy vs. Modern Science

Alchemy, a word that conjures images of shadowy labs and mystical transformations, has roots that stretch back thousands of years. Ancient alchemists sought the elusive Philosopher's Stone, believed to grant the power to transmute base metals into gold and provide the secret to immortality. While these pursuits may seem like fanciful myths today, the practice of alchemy was more than just a quest for material wealth. It was a precursor to modern chemistry, driven by a profound curiosity about the nature of matter and life.

In the modern world, science has unraveled many of the mysteries that alchemists strained to understand. We now know that the transformation of one element into another involves nuclear reactions and that immortality remains beyond the reach of human technology. However, the essence of alchemy—its quest for the potential within substances—persists in contemporary scientific inquiries. Alchemists' holistic approach and belief in a relationship between the spiritual and the physical resonate with some of today's discussions on integrative medicine, which aims to combine traditional healing with modern science.

Alchemy's Legacy: Foundations of Chemistry

The transition from alchemy to chemistry represents one of history's most profound paradigm shifts. Modern scientists stand upon the work of early chemists, who were themselves deeply influenced by alchemical practices. The meticulous methods and observational skills honed by alchemists served as an informal breeder pool for what would eventually become methodologies used in empirical research and the formulation of scientific laws.

Robert Boyle, often hailed as a father of modern chemistry, was among those who helped bridge the gap from mysticism to rationality. His publication, "The Sceptical Chymist," challenged some of the era's prevailing alchemical views and highlighted the importance of observation and experimentation, solidifying chemistry's scientific basis.

Yet, despite its bare bones apparent today, alchemy was not entirely devoid of scientific merit. Alchemists laid the groundwork for techniques such as distillation, extraction, and calcination, which remain fundamental to chemical practices. This intersection between spiritual belief and empirical observation contributed significantly to the toolset of modern chemistry. *In this blend of science and mystery, we uncover the alchemists' true legacy—the spirit of inquiry.*

Ancient Remedies: Precursor to Modern Pharmacology

Alchemical practices were not restricted to metallurgy and philosophy. Many alchemists acted as proto-pharmacists, creating elixirs and remedies that served as precursors to today's medicines.

These early attempts at "medical alchemy" reflected a nascent understanding of chemistry as a means for healing.

Medicinal concoctions of the time, often based on plants, minerals, and metals, were used to treat a wide range of ailments. While experimental and sometimes perilous, these practices embody the early trial and error essential to medical advancements. Some alchemical principles, such as the balancing of bodily humors, can be seen to foreshadow modern notions of homeostasis and physiological balance.

Today, scientific investigations continue to derive insights from historical texts, teasing apart the empirical from the mystical using advanced analytical techniques. The tools of modern science allow for a nuanced understanding and potential rediscovery of bioactive compounds from these ancient formulas. This curious dialogue between past and present prompts an appreciation for how far medical science has advanced, yet urges us to consider what else might be gleaned from ancient teachings.

Transformation: A Metaphor in Medicine

The alchemical idea of transformation finds resonance in modern medical research, particularly within the realm of cancer therapies, genetic engineering, and regenerative medicine. The concept of transforming one's physiological or genetic makeup evokes the alchemist's faith in transmutation. Medicine today continues its quest to fundamentally change the body's state of health.

The symbolic transformation from lead to gold parallels the therapeutic journey from illness to wellness. This allegorical process becomes all the more striking as scientists work tirelessly to change cellular environments to eliminate disease and optimize body functions. This transformation doesn't escape the influence of imagination—the same imagination that inspired alchemists centuries ago.

Indeed, innovation often owes its inception to the visionary pursuit of what lies beyond current understanding. In this quest for change, the lines separating ancient alchemical philosophy from modern scientific practice blur, highlighting a shared determination to push the boundaries of what is possible.

Holistic Intersections of Mind and Matter

Alchemy's philosophical dimensions, which entwine spiritual and physical transformation, reverberate through modern explorations of the mind-body connection. Historically, alchemists adhered to a worldview that emphasized the unity of mental and physical health, a notion gaining traction in contemporary integrative medicine.

This holistic perspective views the body as more than just a collection of biological processes. Instead, it recognizes the influence of psychological states on physical well-being, and vice versa. Today's researchers probe into the psychosomatic intersections that alchemists intuited centuries ago, exploring how stress, thought patterns, and emotional well-being impact bodily health via measurable biochemical pathways.

By redefining health in more comprehensive terms, modern science taps into an alchemical wisdom—one that appreciates the interrelatedness of life's elements. In cultivating such connections, researchers aim to foster solutions that embrace the totality of the human experience in pursuit of optimal health.

Reconciling the Mystical and the Empirical

While alchemy and modern science diverge in their methodologies and mindsets, their shared journey speaks to the enduring human quest for knowledge. Both disciplines strive to unlock the secrets of the universe and the intricacies of health, albeit through different languages and explanations.

Today's scientific advancements have provided answers to questions the alchemists could merely pose. Yet, modern researchers continue to face complex questions that challenge the boundaries of current understanding, echoing the alchemists' adventurous spirit. The historical interplay between alchemical philosophies and the evolution of science invites reflection on humankind's intellectual progression and shared drive to discover.

In acknowledging these intersections, we can more deeply appreciate how ancient alchemy's blend of mysticism and inquiry laid the groundwork for scientific exploration today. Though the language has changed, the spirit of investigation and wonder lives on, urging us along new pathways in the ceaseless journey of discovery.

Alchemical Practices in Healing

Alchemy, often shrouded in mysticism and associated with the arcane quest to turn base metals into gold, also holds a lesser-known connection to healing practices. In historical narratives, the alchemist's lab was not just a place of magical transformations but a hub of medicinal experimentation. Ancient alchemical practices laid the groundwork for many modern pharmaceuticals and holistic treatments, bridging the gap between metaphysical aspirations and tangible medicinal benefits.

In the heart of alchemical practices, the use of plants, minerals, and metals played a significant role in treating various ailments. Alchemists believed that every material had an intrinsic essence that could be harnessed for healing. This belief was not simply philosophical; it reflected a sophisticated early understanding of elemental properties. While the methodologies might seem outdated to the contemporary scientific mind, they introduced concepts that are still relevant today, such as the interaction of different substances within the body.

A cornerstone of alchemical medicinal practices involved the preparation of "spagyric" remedies. This process, which included the separation, purification, and recombination of substances, echoes the pharmaceutical processes used in modern medicine. The spagyric method aimed to extract the vital essence of a plant or mineral to enhance its efficacy. This echoes the modern-day extraction of active ingredients from natural sources to create potent medications.

The art of alchemy wasn't just concerned with the physical. Alchemists also believed in the alignment of the mind, body, and spirit, a precursor to today's holistic health approaches. This holistic view is what makes alchemical healing practices particularly intriguing to those interested in alternative medicine. The notion that physical health is interconnected with emotional and spiritual well-being continues to influence many contemporary holistic healing modalities.

One of the most intriguing alchemical practices is the preparation of elixirs and tinctures. Alchemists aimed to create substances that not only cured but revitalized the body. These concoctions were early forerunners to modern vitamins and supplements. They often sought to restore balance and health by introducing missing elements identified through an intuitive understanding of bodily needs. The search for the "Elixir of Life" symbolizes the perpetual quest for optimal health and longevity that continues to this day.

The synergy between alchemical practices and contemporary science is evident in the ongoing exploration of metals such as gold and selenium in medical treatments. Alchemists considered metals as carriers of essential properties which could be used, albeit with caution, to heal the body. They believed in the transformative power of these metals, a concept that invites parallels to current ideas about oxidative stress and metalloproteins in biological systems.

Despite the mystical aura enveloping these practices, alchemy introduced methodologies that bore surprising resemblances to empirical study. Alchemists relied heavily on observation and trial-and-error, foundational techniques of scientific inquiry. The distinction, however, lay in their approach, which was as much art as it was science. This fusion of creativity with experimentation can often pave the way for breakthroughs in fields that appear stagnant.

The story of alchemical practices in healing is incomplete without mentioning the spiritual component, often embedded within rituals and philosophy. Alchemists advocated for meditative practices and the purification of the soul, emphasizing that effective healing was inseparable from individual transformation. While contemporary medicine often separates physical treatment from mental health and well-being, many alternative practitioners advocate for a return to this more integrated view.

The challenge today is to discern the useful from the mythical in these historical practices. While alchemy is steeped in symbolism and mysticism, the persistence of its principles in modern health approaches demonstrates their enduring relevance. There's a growing interest in rediscovering these practices, not as literal truths but as insights into the interconnectedness of body and nature.

What can we learn from alchemical healing? Perhaps its most valuable lesson is the recognition of healing as an art as well as a science. By blending empirical evidence with holistic health principles, we can better address the complexities of human health. Recognizing this can broaden the scope of medical practice, making room for both rigor and creativity, hopes and clinical evidence, where old wisdom meets new understanding.

In summary, alchemical practices in healing are as much about the process as they are about the substances used. They taught early practitioners to look for deeper connections within nature's myriad elements and to seek balance and transformation as part of the healing journey. These ancient insights continue to inspire modern health disciplines, encouraging a more exploratory and inclusive approach to healing.

Chapter 4: Gold and Cancer Treatment

In the intricate sphere of cancer treatment, gold's inclusion poses both a promise and a puzzle, capturing the curiosity of researchers and clinicians alike. With its unique properties, gold nanoparticles have emerged as a focal point in oncological studies, aiming to revolutionize how we perceive treatment efficacy and safety. They've been implicating in enhancing drug delivery and improving the precision of therapeutic targeting, but the science isn't without its skeptics. Critics voice concerns over long-term toxicity and ethical implications, drawing attention to the necessity for rigorous clinical trials. Patient anecdotes abound with tales of recovery and resilience, providing a narrative rich in hope but fraught with the complexities of placebo effect and subjective reporting. As researchers examine these perspectives alongside hard clinical data, the task becomes one of balancing optimism with scientific rigor, ensuring that gold's potential doesn't overshadow patient safety and realistic expectations.

Examining Clinical Studies

In the complex realm of cancer treatment, gold has emerged as a surprising protagonist. While its use may sound unconventional, the allure of gold in cancer management is rooted in a series of clinical studies that have generated considerable interest and debate. The potential of gold compounds to serve as a therapeutic agent against cancer isn't a recent discovery, but the execution of modern clinical studies has illuminated its possible mechanisms and effects.

The scientific journey to understand gold's impact on cancer involves numerous studies, each contributing pieces to a puzzle that is far from complete. Understanding these studies requires an examination of various factors, including the different types of gold compounds used, their methods of delivery, and the specific cancers targeted. The diversity of approaches reflects the complexity of biological processes involved, and how gold interacts with cancerous cells.

One significant study came from researchers investigating the use of gold nanoparticles. These tiny particles can be engineered to carry chemotherapy drugs directly to cancer cells, potentially sparing healthy cells from damage. The brilliance of this method lies in its targeted approach, aiming to improve the efficacy of treatment while minimizing side effects. This paradigm shift in treatment strategy is one area where gold could redefine traditional chemotherapy approaches.

However, it's not just about how effective gold can be on its own. Many studies focus on its potential role as an adjunctive treatment, working in tandem with existing cancer therapies. For instance, certain gold compounds may enhance the effectiveness of radiotherapy by making cancer cells more susceptible to radiation. This synergistic effect is a promising avenue, showing how traditional and novel treatments can complement each other to better manage cancer.

While the potential is promising, clinical studies also examine the safety profile of gold-based treatments. Researchers are diligently working to understand the toxicological aspects, ensuring that introducing gold into the body will not lead to unforeseen adverse effects. It's a delicate balance: the body must tolerate the treatment while effectively combating cancer cells.

The breadth of clinical studies reflects the diverse opinions within the medical community regarding gold's role in cancer therapy. While some hail the metal as a breakthrough, others call for caution, urging that more data is needed. This divergence is often seen in the results of smaller-scale studies that may show initial promise but lack the robustness of larger, more comprehensive trials.

Another critical aspect scrutinized in clinical studies is the method of administration of gold-based treatments. From orally administered gold salts to intratumoral injections of nanoparticles, methods vary greatly. Each mode of administration comes with its pros and cons, often affecting the absorption rate, distribution within the body, and overall effectiveness.

Notably, the innovative use of gold-based nanotechnology has propelled these studies into the spotlight. Such studies often involve interdisciplinary teams, bringing together oncologists, chemists, and biomedical engineers to explore the possibilities extraordinarily. The flexibility of gold nanoparticles in being modified and functionalized to seek out and target specific cancer cells is a testament to this collaboration among diverse fields.

Despite these advances, skepticism remains. Skeptics often point to inconclusive data or the lack of long-term studies as points of concern. The scientific community is rightly cautious; promising small-scale studies must be backed by large, controlled clinical trials that can demonstrate consistent benefits across diverse patient populations. This highlights the crucial need for peer-reviewed publications and replicability of results.

Currently, one of the hurdles is translating these clinical studies from theory into practice. Cost, regulation, and public perception all play roles in how quickly innovations reach patients. Some studies are still in the early phases, focused on understanding interactions at a cellular level before human trials can be safely conducted.

As we examine these clinical studies, it's clear that gold's potential in cancer treatment isn't a question of if but rather how and when.

With ongoing research and increasing investments, there's hope that more concrete answers will emerge. In navigating these possibilities, the weight of scientific and clinical evidence will ultimately guide practical applications.

In conclusion, the examination of clinical studies reveals a field in flux, driven by curiosity, hope, and rigorous scientific inquiry. While gold as a cancer treatment isn't yet a mainstay, its potential merits a place in ongoing research. These studies hint at a future where gold might contribute significantly to more personalized, effective, and less debilitating cancer treatments. The road ahead requires patience, open-mindedness, and collaboration to fully realize gold's potential in oncology.

Evaluating Patient Anecdotes

When it comes to cancer treatment, stories from patients are like the unscripted moments in a play. They're raw, real, and often seeped in emotions that are hard to capture in clinical research. Listening to these anecdotes can offer unique insights that complement our understanding of how unconventional therapies, such as those involving gold, impact patients.

Among the tales of gold as a cancer treatment, some stand out not for their miraculous claims, but for the poignant human experiences they reveal. Patients report turning to gold, not after being dazzled by wild claims, but often out of desperation as they seek salvations that mainstream medicine has yet to deliver. The anecdotal evidence surrounding gold's use in cancer treatment contains a variety of outcomes. Stories of improved quality of life exist alongside those that are less promising. These personal narratives demand attention, offering a mosaic of hope, disappointment, and resilience.

But it's not just the claims of outcome that matter; it's the context. Consider the way in which patients describe their journeys with gold treatments. Some have noted increased energy and a stabilization of symptoms. For them, these were not just fleeting improvements but changes that extended the possibilities for remission. Accounts of decreased nausea, better appetite, and enhanced mental clarity have been documented. Yet, skeptics abound, pointing out that such stories can be colored by the placebo effect or temporal coincidences. Straightforward, measurable improvements often juxtapose these lived experiences against a backdrop of uncertainty.

It is crucial for anyone examining these patient anecdotes to appreciate the role of setting. The support systems available — or unavailable — to these patients influence their perceptions. Treatments involving gold often occur outside the confines of typical healthcare environments. These settings can uniquely shape a patient's experience, potentially altering their perception of efficacy and well-being.

Anecdotes also reveal the psychological battles that come with navigating illness. For some, the allure of gold treatments stems less from promises of cure and more from the chance to regain a sense of control over their health. Patients frequently discuss how adopting an alternative treatment approach can bring psychological benefits — a renewal of hope and a reaffirmation of self-efficacy. In the fight against cancer, where the human spirit is tested daily, such mental uplift can be as valuable as any physical improvement.

Critically evaluating these anecdotes requires an understanding of their innate limitations. Patient stories often lack the scientific rigor of clinical trials; they're not double-blinded or placebo-controlled. Yet, dismissing them outright ignores a potentially critical supplement to quantitative data: the qualitative experience of living with cancer. The challenge lies in distilling what elements hold potential value from those narrative details, which might merely cloud the discussion.

Another layer to consider is the community aspect of these anecdotes. Patients sharing their experiences with gold often find solace and camaraderie with others in similar situations. This shared narrative can amplify the feeling of validation and authenticity, even in the absence of scientific endorsement. Such community narratives can crystallize into a form of collective social proof that influences newcomers considering gold therapies.

For medical professionals, these stories serve as a reminder that the medical journey is intensely personal. While anecdotal evidence should never replace medical advice, it can inform patient-doctor conversations, ensuring care is nuanced and empathetic. When patients bring these stories to their doctors, they also bring a request: for understanding, for validation, for treatment that considers more than just cells and pathology but the whole person.

The role of the physician, then, becomes not only that of the healer and scientist but also the listener and interpreter. Whereas empirical data drives practice, these patient stories humanize it, reminding clinicians of the individual seated before them. In many cases, negotiating the chasm between empirical and anecdotal evidence is where the true art of medicine lies.

Thus, evaluating patient anecdotes about gold in cancer treatment is not merely an exercise in validation but an exploration of the human condition confronted with adversity. We must consider these stories alongside clinical evidence, keenly aware of their potential limitations while acknowledging their undeniable resonance. Through this lens, anecdotes become not just stories to be told but elements of a complex narrative that can inform our understanding of gold's role in holistic cancer care.

Chapter 5: Selenium and Cancer Prevention

Delving into the intriguing realm of selenium and its potential role in cancer prevention, we find ourselves navigating a landscape rich with promise and complexity. Scientific insights suggest that this trace element, often found in soil, may possess the ability to guard against certain types of cancer. Selenium acts as a powerful antioxidant, neutralizing harmful free radicals and fortifying our cellular defenses. While the medical community continues to investigate, real-world case studies provide a glimpse into selenium's potential—a few epidemiological studies have hinted at lower cancer rates in populations with optimal selenium levels. Still, it's crucial to remain cautious. The balance of selenium intake is delicate; too little may not harness its benefits, while too much could pose risks. As we gather more evidence, it's clear that selenium might play a pivotal role in preventive strategies, but further research is essential to unlock its full potential without overshadowing its complexities.

Scientific Insights into Selenium's Role

Selenium's role in cancer prevention continues to intrigue researchers, drawing them into a web of promising yet complex biochemical interactions. As science grapples to fully elucidate these dynamics, selenium finds itself at the crux of health discussions, acting as both an essential micronutrient and a potential shield against carcinogenesis. The investigations into selenium's biochemical pathways unveil a tapestry of cellular processes, augmenting our understanding of how this element might stave off cancer in various forms.

One of the more persuasive facets of selenium's influence involves its role as a critical component of antioxidant enzymes, particularly glutathione peroxidases. These enzymes combat oxidative stress, a key factor in DNA damage and the subsequent initiation of cancerous growths. By scavenging free radicals, selenium doesn't just neutralize these volatile elements; it fortifies cellular defense mechanisms, thereby reducing the potential for malignancies to take root. Observational studies have consistently shown that populations with higher selenium levels often report lower incidences of certain cancers, underscoring its significant preventative potential.

In the heart of selenium research lies its dual function: antioxidant protection and modulation of cell cycle processes. Selenium's influence extends into the realm of cellular apoptosis—programmed cell death—and inhibits cellular proliferation, both critical in preventing the uncontrolled growth that defines cancer. Proteins like selenoproteins play a commanding role here, intervening in molecular pathways that might otherwise lead to tumorigenesis. This insight shifts selenium from mere nutrient status to that of a molecular custodian, maintaining cellular integrity and balance.

The epidemiological backdrop of selenium and cancer reveals nuanced relationships between selenium status and cancer risk. For instance, studies have shown correlations between low selenium levels and increased risks of prostate, lung, and colorectal cancers. However, selenium's influence doesn't exhibit uniformity across all cancer types, suggesting a complex interplay influenced by genetic, environmental, and dietary factors. Such discoveries compel researchers to investigate selenium's site-specific actions and how it synergizes with local biochemical environments.

Beyond its general antioxidant activity, selenium's activity seems to engage particular molecular pathways that might elicit cancer protection. The role of selenium in the modulation of gene expression, particularly in enhancing tumor suppressor genes and repressing oncogenes, offers another avenue of investigation. By directly interacting with the DNA, selenium can potentially alter the course of cellular differentiation and maturation, reducing the likelihood that cells will deviate into malignant paths.

Various studies, including interventional trials, have provided conflicting yet intriguing results concerning selenium supplementation and cancer prevention. For instance, the Nutritional Prevention of Cancer (NPC) trial initially highlighted selenium's promise against non-melanoma skin cancer but suggested extended benefits for prostate cancer among men. Nevertheless, further large-scale studies like the Selenium and Vitamin E Cancer Prevention Trial (SELECT) provided less optimistic results, raising crucial questions about effective dosages and potentially differing impacts based on selenium's form and bioavailability.

Hence, formulating an accurate picture of selenium's prophylactic role against cancer necessitates understanding not only biological mechanisms but also the context in which it operates. The bioavailability and type of selenium consumed become critical factors in realizing its full anti-carcinogenic potential. Organoselenium compounds, for example, such as selenomethionine, appear to possess diverse physiological and pharmacological properties, each warranting sophisticated investigation to unlock their health benefits.

Importantly, researchers are delving into the genetic aspect of selenium responsiveness. Genetic variations, particularly in selenoprotein genes, appear to modify individual responses to selenium, painting a more personalized approach to understanding this element's role in cancer prevention. With genomic technologies advancing, researchers anticipate more comprehensive, possibly tailor-made dietary recommendations that align with individual genetic profiles to optimize selenium's preventive capabilities.

While the theoretical framework describing selenium's protective measures offers a promising blueprint, practical applications need to tread cautiously. The potential toxicity of excessive selenium makes dosage an essential consideration. The fine line between sufficient and harmful selenium intake accentuates the necessity for informed, evidence-backed supplementation guidelines, especially when considered for cancer prevention.

Despite the inconclusive results from some trials, the quest for a comprehensive understanding of selenium's role in cancer prevention persists. The pursuit resembles a mosaic, where varied scientific revelations piece together to form a more complete picture of selenium's biological impact. As research continues, the anticipation remains that ongoing studies will reconcile discrepancies in existing data, thereby forging clearer pathways for selenium's application in preventive healthcare.

In summation, selenium represents an intriguing frontier in oncological prevention research. Scientific insights have begun to chart the contours of its activity amidst the labyrinthine maze of cellular processes. Yet, as researchers refine their methodologies and broaden their scope from molecular biology to genomics, they edge closer to harnessing selenium's full, preventive promise. Whether through tailored nutritional advice or nuanced therapeutic strategies, the potential for selenium to play a substantive role in human health remains a chapter still unfolding.

Real-World Case Studies

In recent years, the interest in selenium's potential for cancer prevention has seen a marked increase, spurred by both scientific inquiry and anecdotal evidence. To fully appreciate the depth of selenium's impact in real-world scenarios, it's crucial to examine case studies that not only highlight successful outcomes but also underscore the complexities involved in interpreting these narratives within the broader context of cancer prevention.

Consider a pivotal case involving a large-scale study conducted in a rural area of China, where selenium deficiency was prevalent. Researchers implemented a community-based intervention to supplement the population's diet with selenium. Over a period of several years, they observed a decline in the incidence of liver and esophageal cancers, which were once predominant in the region. This case illustrates the potential role that environmental and dietary factors can play in modulating cancer risk, though it also raises questions about the specificity of selenium's protective effects and the interplay of other nutritional variables that may have contributed to the observed health outcomes.

Another compelling case study can be found in the archival data of the Nutritional Prevention of Cancer (NPC) trial, which was conducted in the United States. This randomized study aimed to determine the efficacy of selenium supplements in preventing nonmelanoma skin cancer among individuals with a history of basal cell or squamous cell carcinomas. The findings were intriguing: while selenium didn't significantly reduce the risk of skin cancer, participants receiving selenium supplements exhibited a marked decrease in the overall incidence of prostate cancer.

The NPC trial's insights pivotally shifted the focus of selenium research towards prostate health. These results ignited further investigations and fueled academic debates about the mechanisms through which selenium could influence carcinogenesis. Despite the promising data, subsequent studies, including the Selenium and Vitamin E Cancer Prevention Trial (SELECT), would later yield mixed findings, prompting a reevaluation of selenium's role in cancer prevention. The interplay of these studies demonstrates the importance of robust methodological designs and the need for cautious interpretation of findings, especially when translating them into public health recommendations.

Beyond the realm of controlled clinical trials, individual anecdotes and case reports often add layers of human experience to the scientific discourse. One such narrative involves a middle-aged man diagnosed with early-stage prostate cancer. Faced with a dilemma between conventional treatment and watchful waiting, he opted for a regimen that included selenium as an adjunctive therapy. After regular monitoring, his medical records showed a stabilization of cancer markers, although attributing his clinical improvement solely to selenium demands a careful consideration of confounding factors, such as his overall lifestyle changes and genetic predispositions.

Such real-world examples also highlight the necessity for personalized medicine approaches in the future application of selenium in cancer treatment. Not all populations and individuals respond uniformly to selenium supplementation, which raises the question of genetic predisposition and selenium metabolism differences influenced by both inherent biology and geographical diet variations.

In yet another instance, healthcare systems in regions with lower selenium soil content have started integrating dietary assessments and supplementation protocols into routine cancer care services. For example, clinics in parts of Finland, where selenium-rich soil is lacking, began collaborating with nutritionists to incorporate selenium-enriched foods into patients' diets. Anecdotal feedback from participants has often mentioned improvements not only in cancer markers but also in general well-being and energy levels. Nonetheless, these observations remain primarily anecdotal without controlled variables for rigorous scientific validation.

It's essential to scrutinize these narratives with a critical eye, especially when alternative medicine claims proliferate online. The advent of social media has amplified personal stories about selenium's benefits, though these accounts often lack the clinical rigor necessary to draw generalized conclusions. While some individuals may report enhanced health outcomes after adopting selenium supplementation, these cases could be influenced by a myriad of factors outside selenium's pharmacodynamic properties.

Despite the enthusiasm and promise reflected in these case studies, there's a clear consensus within the scientific community about the need for continued research. Advanced methodologies, including genetic profiling and comprehensive nutritional studies, could pave the way for more personalized and accurate assessments of selenium's role in cancer prevention. By unraveling the complex interaction between selenium, genetics, and other dietary elements, researchers aim to develop refined guidelines that could benefit at-risk populations more optimally.

The tapestry of selenium's real-world applications in cancer prevention thus remains vibrant and complex. It's defined by the convergence of statistical data, personal experiences, and clinical insights. While these case studies have cultivated a platform of hope and ongoing inquiry, they also underscore the importance of treating each patient's journey as singular and nuanced, urging practitioners and researchers alike to remain both hopeful and critically engaged in their exploration of this fascinating micronutrient. As we continue to unravel selenium's mysteries, the question remains: How can we harness its potential to universally enrich human health while acknowledging the limits and challenges inherent in such endeavors?

Chapter 6: Synergistic Potential of Gold and Selenium

In the exploration of gold and selenium, their potential synergy in health applications stands as a compelling chapter. When these two elements unite, it's not merely a sum of their individual properties but rather a potent interaction poised to enhance therapeutic outcomes. Delving into the world of biochemical interactions, researchers have been intrigued by how gold can amplify selenium's antioxidant capabilities, offering a robust defense against cellular damage. Conversely, selenium might stabilize and potentiate gold's functions, driving interest in their combined use in treatments, especially in oncology. Across various case studies, individuals who've integrated these elements into their health regimens report promising results, especially in enhancing vitality and potentially supporting cancer therapies. While still an evolving area of study, the growing body of evidence suggests that the fusion of gold and selenium might just play a pivotal role in future medical protocols, weaving a narrative of past alchemic dreams meeting modern scientific validation.

Biochemical Interactions Explored

In the realm of alternative medicine, the intricate dance of biochemistry reveals pathways that may hold the key to novel treatments and health benefits. Exploring the synergistic potential of gold and selenium, we are at the cusp of understanding how these two elements interact within the human body. It is not merely about their individual benefits, but rather the unique biochemical interplay that occurs when these elements are combined. Their interactions could unlock transformative approaches for improving health outcomes through unexpected synergies.

Gold, in its monoatomic form, is shrouded in a mystique that stretches back to alchemical traditions. Modern science has only begun to unravel its complexities, moving beyond mere historical curiosities to investigate its potential in contemporary medicine. We know that gold nanoparticles can have unique properties that differ significantly from their bulk counterparts. This discrepancy in properties is key to understanding its role in medical applications, particularly when used alongside selenium, another element boasting a rich medicinal history.

Selenium, an essential micronutrient, plays crucial roles in human physiology. It acts as a cofactor for enzymes involved in antioxidant protection and thyroid hormone metabolism. The biochemical pathways involving selenium are themselves dynamic, influencing immune function and offering protective benefits against oxidative stress. But it is when selenium joins forces with gold that an array of potential biochemical interactions emerges, opening doors to therapeutic advancements.

This synergy could be due to several factors, including their complementary antioxidant properties. Gold's anti-inflammatory effects may complement selenium's antioxidant activities, potentially mitigating cellular stress more effectively than each element could on its own. This interaction could provide a compounded defense, offering enhanced protection against chronic conditions associated with oxidative damage.

Beyond oxidative stress, the potential benefits of the gold and selenium combination lie in their impact on cellular signaling pathways. Studies have shown that selenium can modulate cellular signaling related to apoptosis, or programmed cell death. When combined with gold's potential ability to alter cellular behavior, this duet might influence cancer cells' propensity to undergo apoptosis, paving the way for innovative cancer therapies. Moreover, these interactions might not only affect cancerous cells but also contribute to maintaining cellular homeostasis in healthy tissues.

Looking deeper, the interaction of gold and selenium could engage molecular pathways related to immune response. Selenium's role in enhancing immune function is well-documented, and the inclusion of gold could further bolster this effect. There is evidence to suggest that the two might work together to fine-tune immune activity, optimizing it for both defensive and regulatory roles. This could be particularly beneficial in autoimmune disorders, where modulating the immune response is key.

Another compelling aspect of their interaction involves enzyme modulation. Gold has been shown to inhibit specific enzymes associated with disease processes, while selenium acts as a cofactor for a range of enzymes crucial for maintaining metabolic balance. If these elements influence enzyme activity synergistically, they could open avenues for metabolic regulation that have yet to be fully explored. This coordination could provide insights into managing metabolic disorders at a biochemical level, achieving harmony in bodily functions.

While speculative, the possibility that gold and selenium could interact with gut microbiota warrants exploration. The gut plays a pivotal role in modulating various physiological processes, and any factor influencing microbiota could have broad health implications. Given selenium's known effects on gut health and gold's emerging role in influencing microbial populations, their combined effects could revolutionize how we approach gut-related conditions. We might envisage a scenario where their synthesis results in a favorable balance of gut flora, improving gastrointestinal health and amplifying systemic well-being.

However, unravelling these biochemical interactions is not without challenges. The intricacies of human biochemistry require meticulous research and an interdisciplinary approach that bridges molecular biology, pharmacology, and clinical studies. Each step forward must be validated by scientific scrutiny, ensuring that optimistic hypotheses are grounded in empirical evidence. This involves not just exploring the interactions themselves but understanding how they manifest in different physiological contexts, which is crucial for translating such findings into practical applications.

As we delve into these biochemical interactions, it's crucial to maintain a balanced perspective. While the potential benefits are compelling, they must be weighed against the complexity of biological systems. What works in theory or in controlled settings might face hurdles in real-world applications, where individual variability adds another layer of complexity. The path from bench to bedside requires careful examination to ensure both efficacy and safety.

In conclusion, the biochemical interactions of gold and selenium are a promising frontier in alternative medicine. Their synergy could redefine therapeutic frameworks, emphasizing the importance of understanding elemental interactions within biological systems. As research progresses, we may find that these two elements, when intertwined, offer solutions that neither could provide alone—solutions shaped by the intricate dance of biochemistry. The journey of discovery is ongoing, driven by both curiosity and a commitment to improving human health through innovative and informed approaches.

Case Studies of Combined Effects

Exploring the combined effects of gold and selenium offers a tantalizing glimpse into the intersection of traditional and modern medicine. The alchemical promise of these two elements beckons us to consider possibilities that transcend conventional wisdom. But does this synergy truly exist beyond theoretical speculation? To answer this question, we must dive into the intricate tapestry of case studies that illuminate the real-world impacts of combining gold and selenium in medical applications.

In recent years, researchers have initiated small-scale studies to assess the effectiveness of gold and selenium when used together in therapeutic contexts. One particularly intriguing case involved patients undergoing cancer treatment, where they received complementary doses of both elements. Initial findings suggested that this combination offered a dual protective effect: gold acting as a potential disruptor of tumor growth while selenium bolstered the immune system. Such dual action not only provided an enhanced barrier against cancer progression but also mitigated some of the side effects associated with conventional therapies.

Another case study, rooted in the realm of anti-aging and chronic disease management, highlighted the role of these elements in oxidative stress reduction. Medical professionals administering both elements noted significant improvements in the oxidative biomarkers of participants. The synergy seemed to amplify antioxidant activity, thereby promoting cellular health and reducing degeneration rates. While these results were encouraging, they also raised questions about the appropriate dosing and long-term implications of such treatments, underscoring the need for further investigation.

Perhaps the most compelling stories come from patient testimonials, which bring a personal dimension to the scientific data. Take the experience of a middle-aged woman battling rheumatoid arthritis, for instance. After conventional treatments provided limited relief, her physician introduced a regimen that included gold compounds combined with selenium supplements. Over the course of several months, she reported reduced joint inflammation and greater mobility—an outcome that was both unexpected and transformative. These personal narratives, while anecdotal, often kindle interest in pursuing alternative therapeutic avenues.

Moreover, the neurological benefits from the synergy of gold and selenium have been a focus. In a small study involving patients with early-stage Alzheimer's disease, researchers observed a noticeable delay in cognitive decline when both elements were administered simultaneously. Though the sample size was limited and the study's duration relatively short, the findings offered a glimmer of hope for developing adjunctive treatments aimed at neuroprotection. Such preliminary data ignite further interest and investigation into the potential for these elements to provide neurological benefits.

However, not all case studies report such unequivocal success. Some documented instances demonstrated minimal benefits or, in rarer cases, adverse reactions. These outcomes emphasize the complexity of employing elemental therapies, where individual responses can vary radically. The inconsistent results highlight a critical need for personalized medicine approaches, where genetic, environmental, and lifestyle factors are considered to optimize the integration of gold and selenium.

In addition to clinical studies, animal models have also been instrumental in understanding the biochemical synergy between gold and selenium. Laboratory studies on rodents, for example, have shown promising results in areas like inflammation control and metabolic regulation. These models provide a controlled environment to dissect the pathways through which these elements exert their effects. Although animal studies don't always translate perfectly to human biology, they serve as an invaluable tool for mapping the landscape before advancing to human trials.

Beyond the laboratory and clinic, the ethnomedicinal practices of various cultures also offer insights into the potential of gold and selenium. Traditional Chinese and Ayurvedic medicines have long revered these elements for their unique properties. Case studies documenting the practices of these cultures give us a historical context, suggesting a wisdom that's only recently being corroborated by scientific inquiry. These accounts inspire a dialogue between ancient knowledge and modern validation, leading us to reevaluate our approaches to healthcare.

As we sift through these case studies, we are reminded of both the promise and challenges inherent in synergistic therapies. While the positive outcomes inspire enthusiasm, they accentuate the pressing need for rigorous research to substantiate anecdotal evidence with empirical data. Integrating these elements into healthcare regimens requires careful consideration of their interactions with other treatments, patient-specific factors, and long-term effects.

In conclusion, the case studies of gold and selenium, when combined, paint a picture that is at once hopeful and cautionary. They urge us to continue exploring the frontiers of what is possible in alternative and integrative medicine. With each study, we take a step closer to understanding not just the potential of these elements, but the intricacy of their interactions within the human body. The journey from anecdote to evidence is long, but it's a path worth navigating for the potential it holds in transforming medical practice. While definitive conclusions may still be on the horizon, these cases compel us to keep searching, testing, and learning.

Chapter 7: The Controversy of Alternative Treatments

In the realm of alternative treatments, controversy often takes center stage, sparking debates that compel us to question the very nature of healing. Critics argue these treatments stray too far from conventional scientific methodologies, raising the specter of skepticism among medical professionals. Yet, proponents see potential in these unconventional paths, championing their holistic appeal and anecdotal successes as indicators of untapped healing power. This dichotomy creates a tension that becomes a fertile ground for both new ideas and skepticism, urging us to explore these treatments with a discerning eye. While traditional medicine excels in proving efficacy through rigorous clinical trials, alternative treatments often rely on historical wisdom and personal testimonials that challenge our understanding of health and wellness. As we delve deeper, the key lies in addressing criticisms with evidence and openness, fostering a bridge between age-old wisdom and modern science. This balanced perspective not only informs readers but also emboldens them to make educated decisions about their health journeys.

Understanding Skepticism

The world of alternative treatments is as vast as it is controversial, and one can't delve into it without confronting skepticism. This skepticism, like a shadow, trails the promise of alternative therapies at every turn. What's the reason behind such pervasive doubt? To understand this, we must first acknowledge that skepticism in medicine, both conventional and alternative, often stems from a quest for evidence and a need for reliable outcomes. However, the road to acceptance and understanding is fraught with complexities.

In the realm of alternative treatments, skepticism doesn't simply arise from a disregard for innovation or new treatments. It's rooted in historical experiences where the promise of breakthroughs either didn't materialize or resulted in unexpected outcomes. The scientific community, by and large, operates within a framework of rigorous validation, dependent on empirical evidence and reproducibility. These criteria are often where alternative treatments appear to falter, predominantly because many have not been tested through conventional processes due to a lack of funding or the challenges inherent in studying such dynamic and individualized approaches.

Even so, it's crucial to consider that skepticism is not inherently negative. It's a vital part of scientific progress and medical advancement. Skepticism prods us to question, to test, and to demand proof. Any treatment, regardless of its origins or popularity, must stand up to scrutiny to be considered viable or dependable. For alternative treatments, the lack of randomized controlled trials and peer-reviewed studies often fuels this doubt. These treatments can sometimes appear under-researched, especially when compared to conventional medicine.

Moreover, personal anecdotes and patient testimonies that many alternative treatments rely on are often viewed with caution. Doctors and medical professionals see these accounts as the starting point for further investigation rather than evidence of efficacy. While stories of success can be compelling, the scientific community upholds that anecdotal evidence is not a substitute for scientific data. Without controlled conditions and statistical analysis, these narratives remain, at best, inspirational prompts that demand further inquiry.

However, science itself is not infallible. Conventional medicine, though backed by rigorous testing, has its own share of setbacks, historical examples of significance where treatments once thought safe were later deemed harmful. This isn't to undermine the credibility of established practices but to highlight that skepticism must be evenly applied. For alternative treatments, it's about finding a balance between being open to possibilities and demanding assurances about safety and efficacy.

The issue of skepticism in alternative treatments is further complicated by the pharmaceutical industry's role in medical research and practice. There's a perception that economic motives sometimes overshadow the quest for truth. New, potentially effective treatments, especially those not easily patented or monetized, may not receive the attention they deserve. This economic factor can color skepticism, prompting a more critical examination of who's funding and benefiting from the research—or lack thereof.

This skepticism isn't just confined to the medical community. Patients and health-conscious individuals also express doubts, often fueled by mixed messages from both mainstream and alternative medicine practitioners. Conflicting reports and a deluge of information available at the click of a mouse mean individuals are left sorting through claims, trying to discern fact from fiction. This task isn't made easier by the rise of online platforms that can amplify both credible and dubious information with equal fervor.

For the medical community to effectively address skepticism towards alternative treatments, clear communication is paramount. It requires not just explaining the gaps in research or the current stance of conventional medicine but also a willingness to engage with the alternatives respectfully and objectively. There's a dire need for more collaborative research efforts that honor the strengths of both conventional and alternative approaches, uniting them where possible for the benefit of patient outcomes.

This bridge-building approach goes hand in hand with educating patients about the nature and origin of skepticism, helping them understand its role and how it serves as a critical tool for distinguishing between promising therapies and unfounded claims. By promoting transparency about ongoing research efforts and findings, healthcare practitioners can foster a greater level of trust and understanding. Patients, in turn, become more adept at making informed choices, equipped with a nuanced comprehension of the multifaceted issues involved.

In conclusion, skepticism, while appearing at odds with the open-mindedness needed to explore alternative treatments, is essential. It's the mechanism that ensures we don't just accept claims at face value, that treatments prove their worth, and that patient welfare remains the ultimate priority. In future chapters, we'll delve into how criticisms are addressed, dissecting where skepticism serves us best and where it might be unnecessarily stifling progress. It's a delicate interplay that continues to shape the evolving landscape of medicine and health. As we move forward, understanding skepticism will guide not just our evaluations but our aspirations for integrating diverse healing practices in a manner that respects tradition, innovation, and above all, human experience.

Addressing Criticisms

Criticisms of alternative treatments often arise from the clash between traditional medical paradigms and emerging, less-documented methodologies. Skeptics argue that such treatments lack sufficient scientific backing, leading to questions about their legitimacy. A deeper examination reveals that these criticisms can stem from a mix of valid concerns and misconceptions, underscoring the need for a balanced discourse.

First and foremost, one of the most prevalent criticisms is the purported lack of rigorous scientific evidence supporting alternative treatments, such as those involving monoatomic gold or selenium. Many detractors point out that anecdotal evidence and small-scale studies do not meet the gold standard of randomized controlled trials. While this is a legitimate concern, it's worth noting that the cost and complexity of conducting large-scale studies can often inhibit progress in validating alternative therapies. This barrier fuels a vicious cycle; without studies, treatments are considered unproven, yet without approval, studies are challenging to fund. Thus, the dialogue needs to shift towards finding practical solutions to this impasse.

Evidently, another significant criticism revolves around the regulatory environment. Critics argue that alternative treatments often operate in a gray area of regulatory oversight, which can lead to inconsistent quality and safety standards. Traditional medicine adheres to strict guidelines, ensuring that interventions are safe and effective. The absence of similar well-defined standards in alternative medicine may cause unease among medical professionals and potential patients. However, some advocate for more inclusive regulatory frameworks that acknowledge the unique challenges and potential benefits of alternative treatments without compromising patient safety.

Moreover, the potential interaction of alternative treatments with conventional medical practices raises alarm. Critics worry that patients may forego proven medical treatments in favor of less substantiated alternatives, which could lead to adverse health outcomes. It's vital to underscore that many proponents of alternative medicine do not suggest abandoning conventional treatments but rather integrating them to enhance healing potential. The notion of integrating treatments, however, requires both camps to engage in open dialogue and collaborative research, fostering a more comprehensive healthcare approach.

To address these criticisms effectively, transparency and education play pivotal roles. Proponents of alternative treatments must strive to present their methods and preliminary findings clearly and honestly. This transparency builds trust and allows for constructive criticism to inform further research and development. Additionally, educating both the public and healthcare professionals about the nuances of alternative therapies can demystify these practices, dispelling myths and reducing skepticism.

Furthermore, patient-centered approaches can also address criticisms. Empowering patients with complete information about possible treatment options, including potential risks and benefits, allows them to make informed decisions. Shared decision-making models, where clinicians and patients work together to weigh the evidence and individual preferences, can help mitigate concerns about patients prematurely opting for unproven alternatives.

Financial interests can't be ignored in this discussion. Critics sometimes argue that the promotion of alternative treatments might be driven more by profit than genuine efficacy. This skepticism is hardly unwarranted, given that both traditional and alternative medicine industries are not immune to such influences. It's crucial, therefore, for practitioners and supporters of alternative treatments to maintain ethical standards, ensuring that financial motivations do not overshadow the primary goal of patient well-being.

Another angle to consider is the broader context of health and wellness in which alternative treatments are positioned. Many individuals turn to alternative methods out of dissatisfaction with conventional medicine, which can sometimes feel impersonal or overly focused on specific symptoms rather than holistic health. Acknowledging and addressing the preferences and experiences that drive people towards these treatments can foster greater understanding and potentially bridge gaps between traditional and alternative medicine.

A subset of critics focuses on the cultural aspects of alternative treatments. Some argue that the Western medical model tends to dismiss traditional practices rooted in diverse cultural contexts, potentially ignoring valuable insights. This dismissal not only limits the spectrum of exploration but can also be perceived as a form of ethnocentrism. Encouraging cultural sensitivity and inclusivity in research and practice may pave the way for novel discoveries and a richer understanding of health.

Additionally, while some practitioners of alternative medicine are criticized for lack of formal medical training, it's essential to note a growing trend towards certification and professional education in these fields. Formal training programs, credentialing, and ongoing education can enhance the legitimacy and safety of alternative practitioners, which in turn might alleviate some criticism.

In a complex and evolving healthcare landscape, it's vital to keep questioning and challenging the efficacy of both conventional and alternative treatments. Criticisms should not solely be seen as roadblocks but rather as opportunities to refine practices, subject claims to scrutiny, and ultimately improve patient care. Constructive criticism fosters a culture of continuous improvement, pushing both traditional and alternative medicine towards more effective solutions.

In sum, addressing the criticisms of alternative treatments requires a multi-faceted approach, combining scientific rigor, open dialogue, patient education, ethical practices, and cultural sensitivity. By fostering collaboration, transparency, and mutual respect among all stakeholders in the healthcare ecosystem, we can create a more integrated and patient-centered approach to health and healing.

Chapter 8: Scientific Research Methodologies

In the realm of alternative medicine, where skepticism often overshadows promise, a robust understanding of scientific research methodologies becomes crucial. The validity of clinical trials, the foundation upon which scientific truth stands, needs careful scrutiny and transparent transparency. Analyzing these trials allows us to discern efficacy from anecdotal success, while the rigorous process of peer review ensures that findings withstand critical interrogation by the scientific community before reaching the public eye. Embracing both qualitative and quantitative research enhances our examination of treatments like monoatomic gold and selenium, casting light on their complex interplay within the human body. As we navigate this intricate landscape, it's essential to distinguish between what truly holds therapeutic potential versus what's simply veiled in traditional lore. Proper methodologies not only advance our understanding but also uphold the ethical standards required in contemporary medicine, bridging the gap between hope and evidence. This chapter aims to explore these methodologies, setting the stage for their significant role in validating or challenging alternative treatments.

Analyzing Clinical Trials

The intricate dance of scientific inquiry is often most palpable in the realm of clinical trials. These trials are the backbone of modern medicine, offering a structured pathway to evaluate new treatments, validate effectiveness, and ensure safety. In the context of alternative medicine and novel treatments, like those involving monoatomic gold and selenium, clinical trials serve not just as a beacon of hope but as a crucible where science and tradition merge.

At the heart of a clinical trial lies its design, meticulously crafted to minimize bias and maximize reliability. Randomized controlled trials (RCTs) are often the gold standard, partitioning participants into distinct groups: one receiving the experimental treatment and another receiving a placebo or the standard care. This design helps isolate the true effects of the intervention from the noise of placebo effects or natural fluctuations in health conditions. Yet, in the realm of alternative medicine, achieving true randomization can be fraught with challenges. Patients may have strong preferences based on beliefs, impacting random allocation and potentially skewing results.

Blinding is another crucial pillar in clinical trials, essential for reducing bias. Double-blind studies, where neither participants nor researchers know who receives the treatment versus the placebo, are ideal. But in trials involving substances with distinct tastes, colors, or side effects—common in alternative treatments—blinding becomes a complex task. Ensuring that neither party can distinguish between the trial arms requires ingenuity in trial design, yet it's vital to preserve the integrity of the findings.

Analyzing Data

The real magic often occurs not during the trial itself but in the data analysis afterward. Here, researchers apply statistical methods to determine whether observed effects are genuine or happenstance. They measure variables like efficacy, dosage, side effects, and overall improvements. However, the data's interpretation can be contentious, especially with treatments like gold and selenium, where outcomes might defy conventional logic. Researchers must tread carefully, separating correlation from causation, acknowledging statistical anomalies, and being alert to potential conflicts of interest.

Moreover, the diversity of trial subjects plays a critical role in the generalizability of findings. Trials need participants who represent the broader population, in terms of age, gender, ethnicity, and health conditions, to ensure that results are broadly applicable. Historically, this has been a weak point, with many trials failing to recruit diverse participants. In alternative medicine, where traditional biases might persist, inclusive recruiting becomes even more imperative.

Yet another layer is the ethical considerations inherent in running clinical trials. Informed consent stands at the forefront, requiring that participants are fully aware of potential risks and benefits before enrolling. The balance between hope and realistic outcomes must be communicated clearly, especially for patients seeking relief from serious illnesses who may view new treatments as a last resort. Ethical review boards play a critical role here, scrutinizing trial protocols to protect participants from undue harm or exploitation.

Challenges and Controversies

Clinical trials for alternative medicine run into unique hurdles that conventional medicine might not face. First, there's the skepticism from the scientific community. Alternative treatments often start with anecdotal evidence rather than animal studies or preliminary lab research, the latter being prerequisites for mainstream drug development. This skepticism can influence funding availability, further constraining the research capacity in this field.

Another challenge is regulatory approval. Governing bodies like the FDA in the United States have stringent criteria for approving trials and subsequent treatment protocols. Interventions involving gold or selenium must demonstrate significant benefits over existing treatments or provide compelling evidence for their unique efficacy. Additionally, establishing standardized dosages for such elements, especially when they carry risks of toxicity at higher levels, is another critical hurdle.

The application of rigorous scientific methods to analyze clinical trials shines a light on alternative treatments' true potential, pacing them against established medical practices. While promising results can pivot public perception and practitioner enthusiasm, it's the peer-reviewed processes that provide the most enduring validation. This cycle of scrutiny encourages transparency and calls for a detailed disclosure of trials, methodologies, data interpretations, and all potential conflicts of interest. Such openness is crucial in addressing the controversies and misconceptions often associated with alternative therapies.

In conclusion, clinical trials are the crucible where new treatments are tested and vetted. In the context of treatments involving monoatomic gold and selenium, these trials do more than just assess efficacy and safety—they bridge the gap between centuries-old practices and modern scientific standards. Amidst ethical dilemmas, daunting regulatory landscapes, and public skepticism, they provide a beacon of rigorous exploration, opening paths toward credible, holistic treatment possibilities.

The Importance of Peer Review

Peer review stands as a cornerstone of scientific research methodologies, serving as a gatekeeper that ensures the integrity and credibility of scholarly work. In the realm of alternative medicine, where enthusiasm and skepticism often collide, peer review plays an even more critical role. As innovative treatments, like those involving monoatomic gold and selenium, rise into the limelight, the impartial scrutiny offered by peer review becomes not just beneficial, but essential.

Understanding why peer review is so pivotal begins with acknowledging the complex landscape of scientific inquiry. Unlike casual observations or anecdotes, scientific research demands a rigorous process that can withstand critical evaluation. Peer review offers a way to filter out biases, errors, and methodological weaknesses that could tarnish the findings. For health-conscious individuals and medical professionals alike, it serves as a reassurance that the information they are relying on has been meticulously vetted by experts within the field.

In the evolving field of alternative medicine, the allure of new treatments often sails ahead of scientific validation. Consider the case of monoatomic gold; its historical allure turns heads, yet we must differentiate historical speculation from scientifically validated efficacy. Peer review acts as a guardian, insisting that any novel claim be substantiated through replicable research before it's accepted as fact. This process not only aids in separating effective treatments from unfounded claims but also protects patients from unproven, and potentially harmful, therapies.

The peer review process typically involves several stages. Once a research study is completed, the findings are submitted to a scientific journal. Here, experts in the field, independent of the research teams, scrutinize the study. They assess the methodology, the statistical analyses, and the conclusions drawn. They consider whether the findings genuinely contribute new knowledge or advancements. If issues are identified, studies may be returned to authors for revisions or, if flaws are substantial, rejected outright. This rigorous approach ensures that only contributions that meet high standards of scientific rigor find their way into the public domain.

However, the peer review process itself is not infallible. Despite its importance, it faces challenges that can impact the quality of reviews and the timing of publication. Sometimes, reviewers may have competing interests or biases that influence their assessment. Moreover, the time-intensive nature of thorough peer review clashes with the rapidly moving pace of medical research. Nevertheless, the strength of peer review lies in its ability to evolve, incorporating measures like blinded review processes and reviewer feedback to continually improve its robustness.

One might argue that the necessity for peer review has never been greater, especially given the ubiquity of information available online. Patients often encounter health claims from less vetted sources, gravitating towards "miracle cures" based on anecdotal evidence rather than scientific consensus. Here, peer review serves as an authoritative voice that demands backing from data and evidence, pushing back against the allure of easy solutions with its rigorous demands for proof.

Take, for example, the application of selenium in cancer prevention. While selenium's role in health is well-documented, its function as a cancer preventative is subject to mixed reviews. Some studies suggest potential benefits, while others show no effect, or even adverse outcomes in high dosages. Without the peer review process to sift through these studies, integrating meaningful interpretations from piles of data could become close to impossible. Through peer review, duplicative studies are encouraged, supporting or refuting these claims, thus incrementally building a clearer picture of selenium's true impact.

Furthermore, peer review extends beyond mere publication. It fosters a culture of critical engagement and continual learning among researchers. By exposing scientists to different perspectives, it encourages a dynamic dialogue that can inspire improvements and inspire new lines of inquiry. This culture is crucial when venturing into the unconventional terrain of alternative medicine, where innovation must be balanced with caution and due diligence.

For medical professionals invested in the credibility of their field, peer review acts as an ally, bolstering evidence-based practice. It also provides a framework for clinical guidelines, informing the treatments prescribed to patients. In alternative treatments that often face scrutiny, peer review can bolster these options with legitimacy, ensuring that those endorsed are those that deliver genuine benefits.

In sum, peer review is not an arcane tradition but rather a dynamic process essential to the progression of sound scientific research. It engenders trust in an era where misinformation can spread rapidly and unchecked. Scientifically, peer review's filtration of proposals and its facilitation of rigorous discussions between experts ensure that innovations in healthcare, including those in alternative medicine, adhere to the highest standards of scientific inquiry. As the realms of alternative medicine and conventional medicine increasingly intersect, the role of peer review becomes ever more significant in solidifying the foundation upon which treatment protocols are built and sustained.

Chapter 9: The Ethics of Alternative Medicine

The application of alternative medicine signifies a delicate balancing act between science and hope, revealing numerous ethical dilemmas along the way. It's a realm wherein decisions are not just rooted in empirical evidence but are also intertwined with personal beliefs and societal pressures. Practitioners must grapple with questions of efficacy and safety, often navigating a rocky terrain filled with enthusiastic proponents and skeptical critics. Here exists a moral responsibility to ensure that treatments do no harm and to present options transparently, without overstating potential benefits. The stakes are high—patients pin their hopes on therapies that may lack extensive scientific backing, raising concerns about informed consent. It's essential to evaluate these practices with rigor while maintaining empathy for those searching for healing outside conventional means. Ultimately, the ethical landscape of alternative medicine demands a conscientious approach that respects patient autonomy while steadfastly adhering to the principles of medical ethics.

Balancing Science and Hope

The realm of alternative medicine often treads a fine line between empirical science and the hope that fuels the pursuit of unconventional remedies. As the boundaries between established medical practices and alternative treatments blur, it's vital to navigate this landscape with both critical eyes and open minds. In the context of alternative medicine, finding the balance between scientific evidence and patients' aspirations can be challenging yet deeply rewarding.

Science relies on rigorous methodology and repeatable results. It demands evidence that withstands scrutiny and often requires significant time to establish. Hope, on the other hand, is immediate and intoxicating. For many patients, especially those who have exhausted traditional options, hope offers a glimmer of possibility. It's the fuel driving them to explore therapies that the mainstream medical community might dismiss.

One pivotal challenge in balancing science and hope lies in the disparity between anecdotal evidence and clinical data. Patient testimonies often shine a light on the potential of alternative therapies, yet these accounts lack the rigorous controls and peer evaluations that characterize scientific research. Doctors and scientists alike urge caution, advocating for a systematic approach. However, the human narrative—rich in personal stories of healing or relief—cannot be entirely discounted.

Additionally, ethical considerations arise when practitioners propose treatments that have not been fully validated through scientific methods. On one hand, there's a moral imperative to offer all possible options to patients in dire situations. On the other, providing hope without evidence opens a Pandora's box of potential exploitation, false promises, and disillusionment. Striking the right balance requires transparency, honesty, and a dedication to the patients' welfare.

For alternative medicine to earn a legitimate place within—or alongside—conventional medical practices, it must embrace the disciplines of scientific research. This isn't merely about credibility; it's about safety and efficacy. Patients deserve to know that their treatments will not only offer solace but also adhere to standards that protect their well-being. It's a call for rigorous trials and conscious pursuit of data that can either substantiate or refute the claims made by alternative practices.

The integration of hope and science is not merely an ideal but a necessity, as patients' faith in their treatment can significantly impact healing outcomes. Studies suggest that belief in treatment— be it traditional or alternative—can activate specific pathways in the brain, bolstering the immune response and enhancing recovery. This mind-body connection hints at why despite lacking scientific rigor, many patients continue to turn to alternative medicine.

Nonetheless, the interpretation of hope should not cloud the critical judgment required for ensuring patient safety. The tension between a patient's right to select their treatment and the responsibility of practitioners to safeguard against unproven remedies is intrinsic to ethical decision-making in healthcare. It's about ensuring that hope does not translate into hazard.

Moreover, cultural contexts can color the perception of alternative treatments, affecting their acceptance in various societies. In some cultures, traditional remedies are deeply rooted in history and identity, lending legitimacy to practices that others might view skeptically. Respecting these traditions while advocating for scientific validation presents yet another layer of complexity in this delicate balancing act.

At the heart of this dialogue is communication. Bridging the gap between healthcare practitioners and patients requires clear, empathetic dialogue. Patients need to be informed participants in their healing journey, aware of both the potential benefits and risks of treatments they might pursue. Doctors and researchers should listen to patient experiences and consider them as valuable data points within a broader research framework.

The convergence of hope and science is not new but rather a persistent theme throughout medical history. Many treatments once considered fringe or experimental are now canonical because they emerged triumphant from the relentless scrutiny of scientific inquiry. Penicillin, once a hopeful speculation, transformed into a cornerstone of modern medicine.

In conclusion, balancing science and hope in alternative medicine requires vigilance, empathy, and a commitment to advancing knowledge for the benefit of all. The journey necessitates courage to challenge the status quo, wisdom to evaluate unorthodox solutions, and patience to allow the slow, deliberate pace of science to unfold. In this convergence lies the potential to innovate the future of healing.

Ethical Dilemmas in Treatment

In the intricate realm of alternative medicine, ethical challenges often emerge as practitioners and patients navigate through treatments outside the conventional medical framework. The crux of these dilemmas lies in balancing hope with empirical evidence, all while ensuring patient safety and informed consent. Alternative medicine, with its myriad forms and philosophies, advocates holistic healing often based on traditional practices, many of which predate modern medical science. This marriage of tradition and innovation calls for a keen ethical inquiry.

One primary ethical dilemma is the question of efficacy versus belief. When treating patients with chronic conditions, or those who feel disillusioned by traditional medical approaches, alternative treatments can offer solace. But therein lies a caveat: the treatment might be rooted more deeply in anecdote than in scientifically validated results. This predicament places both practitioners and patients in challenging positions. They must decipher whether they're pursuing a genuinely effective intervention or simply being buoyed by the placebo effect or wishful thinking.

The issue of informed consent rises prominently in these treatments. Informed consent is a pillar of medical ethics, requiring that patients fully understand the nature and potential risks of the treatment they are about to undergo. With alternative medicine, educating patients becomes more complex. There's often a lack of robust, peer-reviewed studies that patients and practitioners can rely on. This absence of solid scientific grounding can hinder truly informed decisions, raising significant ethical concerns.

Consider also the ethical tensions introduced by financial implications. Many alternative therapies fall outside insurance coverage, compelling patients to bear significant out-of-pocket costs. A treatment's high expense, when contrasted with its uncertain outcomes, may exploit vulnerable individuals desperate for relief. This financial burden isn't merely an economic issue; it comprises an ethical conundrum where the value of relief must be weighed against the tangible cost and risk of exploitation.

Furthermore, the regulatory landscape—or often, the lack thereof—poses another level of ethical complexity. Unlike conventional treatments, alternative medicine frequently operates in a gray area of regulation. This potentially leaves room for practices that might prioritize commercial gain over patient welfare. Without stringent oversight, practitioners can vary widely in their methodology and accountability, thus raising the stakes of ethical practice.

This unpredictability in regulation also complicates the distinction between credible practitioners and those more akin to charlatans. Both may operate under the banner of alternative medicine, but with vastly different motives and outcomes. Without clear guidelines and oversight, it can be challenging to protect patients from those who might be less scrupulous.

Another aspect to consider is the ethical implications of cultural appropriation within alternative medicine. Many alternative treatments are derived from indigenous practices developed over centuries. When these are adopted—or sometimes, adapted—into alternative medicine without respectful acknowledgment, it raises concerns of exploitation. Not recognizing the cultural origins and significance of certain therapies can be ethically problematic, shining a light on deeper issues of respect and authenticity in treatment delivery.

Communication forms the backbone of ethical treatment in alternative medicine, especially given the set of unknowns that inherently accompany it. Effective communication involves not just disseminating information but also being receptive to the patient's beliefs, concerns, and hopes. Practitioners have an ethical duty to engage transparently and compassionately, acknowledging both the limits of their knowledge and the vast unknowns of their practice.

One must also ponder the ethical responsibilities involved in continuing or discontinuing treatment. Practitioners should assess not just the physiological impacts on the patient but also the psychological and emotional ones. The motivation behind a patient's persistence with a particular treatment can sometimes be rooted in the psychological comfort they associate with it, rather than its actual efficacy. Navigating these waters requires sensitivity and integrity, challenging practitioners to weigh benefit against potential harm with utmost care.

Lastly, there's the dilemma of integrating alternative and conventional treatment methods. The synergy between the two could provide holistic health benefits, yet due to differing philosophical foundations, conflicts may arise. How does one ethically employ an alternative treatment without diminishing the patient's compliance with necessary conventional therapies? Should a line be drawn, or is there a way to ethically and effectively merge both approaches?

In questioning the ethical ramifications of treatment within alternative medicine, what surfaces is a broader, enduring question of what constitutes "acceptable risk" in the pursuit of healing. Each treatment, traditional or alternative, whether steeped in scientific corroboration or anecdotal evidence, presents a unique ethical landscape. As practitioners and patients continue this journey together, the navigation of these dilemmas becomes not just an academic exercise but a lived experience. They are the heart of what it means to strive for healing in a world overflowing with information, yet not always with clarity.

Chapter 10: Legal Aspects of Using Alternative Treatments

The realm of alternative treatments sits at a complex junction of hope and regulation, where dreamers and realists face off in the courtroom and beyond. Here, the intricate dance between innovation and legality reveals itself through a web of regulatory challenges and emerging legal precedents. Various agencies, such as the FDA in the United States, have strict protocols that grapple with the unconventional nature of many alternative treatments. Yet, these legal frameworks are often perceived as both a shield for patient safety and a barrier to medical innovation. Over time, notable legal cases have set precedents that either facilitate or hinder the use and acceptance of these treatments. Practitioners and patients alike must navigate this complicated legal landscape, balancing the benefits of alternative therapies against the obligations to comply with existing laws. The stakes are high; decisions in this space can define the accessibility, research, and even the legitimacy of such treatments in the future. As the world moves forward, the ongoing legal battle will play a pivotal role in shaping how alternative medicine integrates with, or stands apart from, conventional medical practices.

Regulatory Challenges

In the rapidly evolving landscape of alternative treatments, navigating regulatory challenges is a complex affair. The world of alternative medicine is marked by both innovation and controversy, where promising new therapies often face intense scrutiny from official bodies. For those advocating for alternative treatments, regulatory frameworks represent both a hurdle and a necessary safeguard.

The regulatory landscape of alternative medicine in countries like the United States is governed by agencies such as the Food and Drug Administration (FDA). The primary aim of such agencies is to ensure that products consumed by the public are safe and effective. Yet, when it comes to alternative treatments, this is easier said than done. The criteria for evaluating traditional pharmaceuticals don't always translate neatly to alternative methods. Factors like biological variability and subjective outcomes complicate standard testing protocols.

A persistent issue is the classification of products. Many alternative treatments, be they herbs, supplements, or less tangible interventions like energy healing, often fall into regulatory gray areas. The categorization of a product can drastically affect the requirements it must meet before entering the market. Is it a food, a drug, or a supplement? Each category carries distinct regulatory hurdles.

Misclassification can lead to products being pulled from shelves or subjected to additional scrutiny, thus delaying public access.

Moreover, the rules governing alternative treatments can vary drastically from one nation to another. This global inconsistency creates challenges for practitioners and companies looking to operate on an international scale. Countries with strict regulatory standards might not recognize certifications from other nations, rendering cross-border sales and international clinical studies complicated endeavors. It's a regulatory maze that can stifle innovation and access to potentially beneficial treatments.

For example, the therapeutic application of gold and selenium, substances with historical roots in alchemy and modern roles in medicine, often brushes up against these regulatory challenges. Both elements are subjects of ongoing research and debate—each claiming health benefits that are difficult to standardize across scientific and anecdotal evidence. The FDA and other similar bodies require extensive clinical trials to substantiate any claims made, which can be prohibitively expensive and logistically challenging for smaller firms and independent researchers.

The cost of compliance is indeed significant and often prohibitive. Conducting the rigorous trials necessary to obtain approval can cost millions of dollars, a burden that can be prohibitive for many smaller companies or research groups dedicated to exploring alternative treatments. This financial strain can act as a deterrent to innovative research and development, potentially leaving promising therapies unexplored.

Then, there's the public perception to consider. Regulatory bodies must tread carefully to avoid stifling innovation while protecting consumers from potential harm. It's a delicate balance. The public, swayed by personal anecdotes and viral stories about miraculous cures, often clamors for quick regulatory approval or, conversely, expresses skepticism toward unexplained scientific endorsements. This creates a unique challenge for those managing the regulatory frameworks, as they must negotiate the fine line between supporting public interest and maintaining scientific integrity.

The regulatory environment is further muddied by legal cases and precedents that can shift the landscape unexpectedly. Class action lawsuits against alternative treatment companies for unsubstantiated claims can have a chilling effect on the industry, pushing firms to become more cautious in their marketing and research assertions. At the same time, successful legal defenses of alternative treatments can set precedents that encourage more open exploration and use of such therapies.

Another layer is added by the ethical implications involved in the regulation of alternative treatments. On one hand, officials must protect patients from false hopes and potentially harmful practices. On the other, they must ensure that regulation does not infringe upon personal liberties or inhibit access to treatments that a patient might wish to explore, especially when conventional options have already been exhausted.

Collaboration between regulatory bodies, researchers, and health practitioners is key in overcoming these challenges. Open lines of communication can facilitate better understanding and clearer guidelines that benefit everyone—from researchers and practitioners to end users seeking alternative treatments. Emerging strategies like adaptive licensing and conditional approvals show promise in creating more flexible regulatory pathways that can adapt to the unique nature of alternative medicines.

Finally, ongoing education for both practitioners and the public remains crucial. By fostering a better understanding of the regulatory landscape—its processes, purposes, and its limitations— stakeholders can work together more effectively. This shared knowledge can promote innovation while safeguarding public health, striking a balance that benefits all parties involved.

Ultimately, navigating the regulatory challenges of alternative treatments isn't just about following rules—it's about evolving those rules to better fit the changing landscape of healthcare. As more people turn toward alternative medicine for health solutions, the need for a robust yet adaptable regulatory framework becomes increasingly essential. The goal is to cultivate an environment where innovation and safety thrive hand in hand.

Legal Cases and Precedents

The increasing popularity of alternative treatments such as monoatomic gold and selenium in health and wellness spheres inevitably brushes against the legal framework designed primarily around conventional medical treatments. This intersection is fraught with complexities, as it raises several legal questions that challenge existing norms and, sometimes, the patience of jurisdictions attempting to keep pace with evolving health paradigms.

One major legal concern involves the marketing and sale of alternative treatments. Several landmark cases have shown how companies often tout these products without adequate scientific backing or with misleading claims about their efficacy and safety. Regulatory bodies like the Food and Drug Administration (FDA) in the United States have historically been cautious, and sometimes resistant, when it comes to approving alternative treatments that lack substantial clinical evidence. A notable case is that of a company selling selenium supplements, which was prosecuted for advertising the product as a cure-all remedy. The court sided with the regulators, emphasizing the necessity for scientific validation in claims made to consumers. Such cases reinforce the need for evidence-based marketing, ensuring that consumers are not misled by unfounded therapeutic claims.

Moreover, the legal landscape is also influenced by the outcomes of malpractice lawsuits concerning alternative treatments. In several instances, healthcare providers have faced legal repercussions after recommending or administering alternative treatments that resulted in adverse effects. Courts have often been tasked with examining whether such treatments met the "standard of care" expected within the medical community. One prominent case that serves as a precedent involved a practitioner who administered monoatomic gold to a patient with terminal illness, claiming it would counteract cancer. When the patient's condition worsened, the family sued, arguing that the treatment was both ineffective and negligently recommended. The court's ruling underscored the obligation of healthcare professionals to adhere to practices that are not only innovative but also backed by reputable scientific research.

Legal precedents also dive into the rights of patients who seek alternative therapies. The principle of patient autonomy supports individuals' rights to choose their treatment paths but does not absolve practitioners from ensuring informed consent. This complex legal battleground often involves discerning whether patients were fully aware of the risks and benefits—often a contentious issue, especially when the alternative treatments in question are not well-documented or understood. Cases across various jurisdictions have highlighted the need for meticulously drafted consent forms and conversations that clearly lay out what patients might expect from these therapies.

The regulatory environment for alternative medicine varies widely across the globe. In the European Union, for instance, the regulation of such treatments is fairly stringent, compelling manufacturers to undergo rigorous assessments akin to those for pharmaceuticals. Hence, legal cases in these regions sometimes hinge on unauthorized sales or distribution rather than practice. For instance, a supplier of alternative treatments was recently embroiled in a lawsuit due to not complying with the European Medicines Agency's regulations, leading to significant penalties and product seizures. This case serves as a cautionary tale about the consequences of ignoring legal statutes, even when global demand and consumer approval might suggest otherwise.

There have also been cases where courts have ruled in favor of practitioners, particularly when alternative treatments are used in conjunction with conventional methods. Such decisions often view the situation holistically, recognizing the potential for alternative treatments to supplement rather than replace traditional processes. An example is seen in a court case where the integration of traditional and alternative treatments was investigated; the ruling recognized the potential benefit to the patient, provided the treatment regimen was well-documented, and the patient was fully informed.

Looking forward, legal precedents in alternative medicine continue to evolve as new treatments and modalities emerge. There's an ongoing tension between innovation in health practices and the inertia of legal systems designed to protect public safety. As research broadens and more case studies become available, courts may adopt a more nuanced understanding of the efficacy and safety of alternative treatments. To that end, case law could become a vital part of the equation, providing guidance for future legal frameworks that balance the necessity for regulatory oversight with a recognition of therapeutic potential.

Ultimately, these legal cases and precedents not only shape the future of alternative medicine but also bring to light the cultural and ethical dimensions of patient care. They stir necessary dialogue regarding how societies value evidence, hope, and the rights of individuals in managing their health. By wrestling with these questions within the courtroom, legal systems contribute to defining the boundaries within which alternative treatments may safely and effectively operate, delineating a path toward integration with conventional medicine in a manner that respects patient choice while safeguarding well-being.

Chapter 11: Case Studies of Recovery

In exploring the spectrum of case studies, riveting tales of recovery unfold, offering a glimmer into the seemingly miraculous potential of alternative medicine. These documented success stories showcase individuals defying the odds through treatments that blend unconventional wisdom with modern medical science. Patients once mired in their ailments find renewed hope; their journeys reflect resilience and determination. What's crucial here is the lessons gleaned from each experience. These narratives don't just bolster anecdotal evidence but also spark compelling discussions in both medical circles and broader communities, provoking thought about holistic healing approaches. Each case study acts as a pivotal lens, highlighting how the intricate dance between patient belief, treatment adherence, and medical guidance can sometimes lead to astounding outcomes. While their success doesn't guarantee universal applicability, the transformational stories invite further inquiry and offer a beacon for those navigating similar health challenges.

Documented Success Stories

Amidst the ongoing debates surrounding alternative medicine, stories of unexpected recoveries have emerged, capturing the interest of both skeptics and proponents alike. These accounts aren't mere anecdotes; they're powerful narratives that reveal the potential of unconventional treatments. Let's delve into some of these documented success stories, where traditional boundaries were challenged, leading to astonishing outcomes.

Take, for example, the case of Jonathan P., a 56-year-old businessman who faced a dire prognosis. Diagnosed with a rare form of cancer, standard chemotherapy offered little hope. Desperate for solutions, Jonathan ventured into the realm of alternative treatments. It was here that he encountered a regimen involving monoatomic gold and selenium supplementation. Under the supervision of both a certified oncologist and a practitioner specializing in integrative medicine, Jonathan embarked on this journey with cautious optimism.

The initial phases were far from smooth. Adjustments in dosage and regular monitoring were crucial. Yet, six months into the treatment, his medical team began noting unexpected changes. Tumor markers, which had been steadily climbing, started to stabilize and eventually decrease. By the end of the year, Jonathan's scans showed significant reduction in tumor size, leaving his conventional doctors astounded.

Jonathan's story isn't an isolated case. Similar narratives echo through support groups and forums dedicated to alternative medicine. Claudia R., a retired school teacher, found herself grappling with debilitating arthritis. Conventional treatments offered limited relief and came with a slew of side effects that impinged on her daily life. Frustrated, Claudia turned towards dietary changes and natural remedies, with a specific focus on selenium due to its anti-inflammatory properties.

Her journey was one of trial and error, but with determination and consistent biofeedback, improvements began to manifest. Within a year, she reported a dramatic decrease in joint pain and an increased range of motion. Her rheumatologist, initially skeptical, had to reevaluate his stance when Claudia's x-rays displayed unexpected joint repair. Instances like these push the boundaries of our understanding and question the status quo.

What makes these cases compelling isn't just the outcome but the process of integration with conventional approaches. Consider the story of a pediatric patient whose story was documented in a peer-reviewed journal. Diagnosed with a severe autoimmune disorder, standard treatments only partially managed the symptoms. When added to his conventional care regimen, a carefully calculated combination of monoatomic elements was introduced, with oversight from medical professionals.

The results were striking enough to be noted in a case study published in a reputable medical journal. Clinical improvement was observed, and long-term follow-ups showed not just symptom management, but indications of remission. This documented case highlighted the potential for collaborative treatment protocols involving both traditional and alternative methods.

However, these stories are not without controversy. Critics argue that they could be outliers or attributed to other variables, like spontaneous remission or placebo effect. The complexity of documenting alternative success stories lies in their deviation from standardized methods. Each case must be evaluated on its own merit, recognizing the intricacies involved.

Nevertheless, these stories serve as powerful reminders of the need for open-mindedness in medical research. They're testament to the evolving landscape of healing and recovery, suggesting that perhaps, the key to success lies in personalized treatment plans that bridge the gap between traditional and alternative methodologies.

Recognizing success stories like these is critical. They inspire further research, not as tales of magical cures but as starting points for scientific inquiry. These documented successes compel researchers to ponder the biochemical interactions at play and the potential mechanisms driving these outcomes. It is in the nature of science to question, to verify, and to expand our collective knowledge.

For medical professionals and health-conscious individuals, these stories provide a constructive dialogue on the merits of integrating diverse modalities into treatment plans. They open the door for further exploration and innovation, urging a reconsideration of what is deemed possible in recovery and health.

Ultimately, these documented success stories invite us into a broader understanding of health, challenging us to venture beyond set boundaries in pursuit of healing. As these narratives continue to unfold, they offer hope and inspiration to those seeking alternative pathways to wellness. The journey of documenting success in alternative medicine is complex and often fraught with tension, but the pursuit of understanding and healing makes it a worthy endeavor.

Lessons Learned from Patients

In the journey of exploring alternative treatments, especially those involving elements like gold and selenium, patients have emerged as some of the most insightful teachers. Across various case studies of recovery, patients have shared their stories, shedding light on both the promise and pitfalls of non-traditional medical approaches. Their experiences offer a rich tapestry of insights that can inform both practitioners and those seeking healing through unconventional means.

An immediate observation from these personal narratives is the profound importance of individualized treatment. Many patients have reported that their successes came not from a one-size-fits-all approach but from treatments that were tailored to their unique biological make-up and health needs. This emphasizes the necessity for personalized medicine, which could mean the difference between progress and stagnation in their healing process.

Moreover, patients' stories highlight the critical role of patient autonomy and involvement in treatment decisions. When individuals are actively involved in their healing journeys, they often report a greater sense of empowerment and, subsequently, improved outcomes. This suggests a paradigm shift where patients are not merely subjects receiving care but are participants in the therapeutic process.

Equally enlightening are accounts related to the psychological and emotional dimensions of healing. Many individuals have detailed how their mental and emotional states significantly influenced their recovery. It turns out that maintaining a positive outlook and having strong emotional support systems were crucial elements that contributed to their overall healing. This reinforces the often-dismissed notion that the mind-body connection can be a powerful ally in recovery.

A recurring theme among patients' experiences is the challenge they faced with skepticism, both internal and external. Interestingly, some patients encountered initial doubt about alternative treatments from their close circles and healthcare professionals. Navigating this skepticism required resilience and, in many cases, a strong belief in their chosen path of treatment. This speaks volumes about the psychological fortitude necessary for those pursuing alternative therapies amidst a primarily conventional medical framework.

Furthermore, patients' anecdotes often mention the value of combining traditional and alternative medicine. Several individuals found success by integrating both approaches, leveraging the strengths of each to enhance their healing. This highlights an opportunity for the medical community to consider hybrid treatment models that respect and incorporate various healing traditions.

From dietary changes to the adoption of lifestyle modifications, many patients have attributed their recovery to holistic approaches that go beyond just treatment with gold and selenium. Dietary adjustments, meditation, and other lifestyle practices have played significant roles in enhancing the efficacy of their treatments. This emphasizes the necessity for comprehensive care strategies that address the multifaceted nature of healing.

On the cautionary side, the experiences of some patients also highlight the potential risks and side effects involved in alternative treatments. While these are extensively covered in separate sections, understanding patients' firsthand experiences serves as a cautionary tale, reminding us of the need for meticulous management of treatments and awareness of possible adverse reactions.

Finally, an invaluable lesson from patients is their ability to adapt and remain hopeful even when faced with setbacks. Many stories are punctuated with tales of resilience, where individuals, despite facing hurdles, continued to persevere, often tweaking their approach and strategy. This adaptability is a lesson in itself - emphasizing that recovery is not always linear and may require persistence and flexibility in approach.

In conclusion, patients teach us that while alternative treatments like those involving gold and selenium hold promise, their real-world application demands consideration of various factors including personalization, psychological support, and integrative practices. As medical professionals and health-conscious individuals alike navigate the landscape of alternative medicine, these lessons from patients serve as both a guide and an inspiration, underscoring the delicate interplay between science, hope, and healing.

Chapter 12: Risks and Side Effects

In navigating the often turbulent waters of alternative medicine, it's crucial to address the potential risks and side effects associated with treatments like those involving monoatomic gold and selenium. Despite their allure and purported benefits, these substances don't come without their share of caveats. Adverse reactions can vary widely, ranging from minor discomforts to significant health concerns, influenced by factors such as dosage, individual health profiles, and existing medical conditions. For health-conscious individuals and medical professionals alike, understanding and managing these risks is paramount to ensuring safety and efficacy in treatment. A keener focus on comprehensive risk assessments not only protects patients but also advances the legitimacy of alternative therapies within the broader medical community. By embracing a careful balance of caution and optimism, practitioners can offer treatments that harmoniously blend evidence-based practices with holistic healing philosophies.

Potential Adverse Reactions

As we journey into the realm of alternative medicine, particularly focusing on the integration of gold and selenium, understanding potential adverse reactions becomes paramount. While the allure of unconventional therapies captivates many, looking at the darker paths they could lead down is crucial for informed decision-making. This chapter seeks to unfold the possible risks that accompany these intriguing treatments.

Monoatomic gold and selenium, individually renowned for their supposed health benefits, also come with a spectrum of reactions not to be taken lightly. With monoatomic gold, for instance, enthusiasts often hail its transformative powers, yet scientific scrutiny reveals a fuller picture. A common concern is its potential neurotoxic effects, despite claims of boosting mental clarity and cognitive function. These effects aren't universally experienced but can manifest in sensitive individuals, raising questions about long-term use.

Similarly, selenium, while essential in trace amounts, can toe a dangerous line if mismanaged. The mineral's role in antioxidant defense and immune function is well-documented, but excessive intake leads to what is known as selenosis. This condition can present with symptoms ranging from gastrointestinal disturbances to more severe complications like respiratory distress and liver damage. This dual face of selenium, thus, necessitates a disciplined approach in its use, especially when leveraged for illness prevention or treatment in high doses.

Interaction between these substances and traditional medications also deserves consideration. Both elements, particularly when used concurrently, can influence or hinder conventional pharmacological actions, potentially yielding unforeseen results. Gold, believed to have anti-inflammatory properties, might alter the effectiveness of medications aimed at similar outcomes. Selenium's antioxidant nature may impact chemotherapy's functionality, as some studies highlight that antioxidants could diminish treatment efficacy.

Moreover, the psychological effects can't be ignored. The promise of alternative treatments often instills hope, yet this psychological investment doesn't come without its risks. The placebo effect can be powerful, making it challenging to discern genuine healing from psychological relief. When treatments don't work as anticipated, the resultant emotional toll can be substantial, leading to feelings of despair or betrayal. These potential adverse reactions are not merely confined to physical health, but extend into the emotional and psychological domains.

Scientifically unverified claims play a significant role in these adverse reactions, as well. The allure of "natural" therapies sometimes seduces individuals into dismissing proven medicinal protocols. With unregulated products, the risk of contamination or inconsistency in dosage exists, and the effects could be unpredictable. Self-administration without professional oversight further compounds these risks, amplifying the potential for harm.

Yet, evaluating the breadth of adverse reactions requires us to acknowledge the subtle balance between benefits and risks. It's common for alternative treatments to promise substantial positive outcomes while underselling potential side effects. Those advocating for or against must present these therapeutic options with caution and transparency. Oversight by health authorities can serve as a critical check, ensuring the proposed benefits of such treatments are reliably vetted and supported by external, unbiased evaluations, potentially curbing the risk of negative outcomes.

In drawing this picture, it's vital to consider genetic predisposition and individual variability. Some might react adversely to what's harmless or beneficial to others. Personalized approaches in treatment protocols are increasingly recognized in mainstream medicine, accentuating the need for such considerations in alternative practices as well. Without personalization, there's a high likelihood of adverse reactions going unnoticed until it's too late. Developing protocols that take an individual's entire health profile into account is not just ideal but essential.

Ultimately, while the potential adverse reactions to monoatomic gold and selenium are a cautionary tale, they remind us of the importance of a careful, balanced approach to health. It's about weighing these risks against the purported benefits, understanding that real healing surpasses quick fixes, and entails a broad consideration of the human body and mind's complex interplays. By respecting this complexity, we not only shield ourselves from potential harm but also pave the path for more informed, possibly revolutionary medical interventions.

Managing Risks in Treatment

Medicine, by its very nature, involves a delicate balance between healing potential and risk. This balance becomes even more complex when integrating alternative treatments, such as those involving gold and selenium, which are explored elsewhere in this text. While many are drawn to these treatments for their promise of benefits, it is critical to acknowledge and manage the potential risks associated with their use.

Firstly, individual variability plays a significant role in how patients respond to any therapeutic intervention. No two bodies are precisely alike, and reactions can differ widely due to factors like genetics, existing health conditions, and concurrent medications. This makes personalized treatment plans a necessity in medical practice, especially when new or unconventional treatments are involved. Practitioners must thoroughly assess each patient's health profile, understand their history, and tailor approaches accordingly to mitigate potential risks.

Another layer of complexity arises from the synergistic use of gold and selenium. While Chapter 6 delves into their combined biochemical interactions, it's vital to recognize that the interaction of these elements might not always yield positive outcomes. Their synergistic potential involves carefully calibrated dosages to prevent adverse effects. Too much of either element could result in toxicity.

Hence, meticulous monitoring and adjustments are imperative throughout the treatment process.

A patient's psychological state is another important consideration. As Chapter 15 discusses the emotional dimensions of healing, it's essential here too. Patients' belief in a treatment can influence outcomes significantly, whether through placebo effects or a genuine psychological link to healing. However, if expectations are not managed appropriately, patients may experience disillusionment or anxiety, detracting from their overall well-being. Open communication between healthcare providers and patients can help manage these expectations and ensure that patients are well-informed about the potential and limits of their treatment options.

Furthermore, understanding and managing risks extend into the realm of healthcare providers themselves. Medical professionals engaging with alternative treatments must remain abreast of current research and developments. Chapter 7 deals with the controversies surrounding such treatments, highlighting the balance between skepticism and open-mindedness. Providers must exercise caution and stay informed to provide accurate, evidence-based guidance while keeping abreast of legal aspects, as noted in Chapter 10.

The regulatory landscape is another critical aspect to consider. Laws and guidelines surrounding the use of alternative treatments vary widely between jurisdictions, and providers must navigate these carefully to ensure compliance and patient safety. This is especially important as legal frameworks evolve to address new treatments and research findings, as detailed later in Chapter 10. Awareness of these legal intricacies helps in managing treatment risks while fostering trust with patients.

Moreover, an essential tool in risk management is ongoing research. As outlined in Chapter 8, robust scientific methodologies, including clinical trials and peer review, provide the foundation for understanding the safety and efficacy of treatments. Continuous research contributes to the dynamic knowledge base that guides practice and aids in the identification and management of potential risks associated with novel therapies.

In practical terms, risk management often boils down to protocols and standard operating procedures. Chapter 19 will further explore how developing safe dosages and using protocols tailored to individual needs can reduce risks. Establishing these protocols ensures consistency in treatment delivery and provides a framework within which healthcare providers can work confidently while minimizing the likelihood of adverse outcomes.

Proactive patient education is another critical component. Patients must be partners in their healthcare journeys, informed about both the benefits and the limitations of any treatment. Health education empowers them to make informed decisions, enhances adherence to treatment plans, and fosters a collaborative relationship with their healthcare providers. Chapter 18 sheds light on strategies for building awareness, emphasizing that informed patients are better equipped to recognize early signs of adverse reactions and seek timely intervention.

Lastly, integrating traditional and alternative medicines, as briefly handled in Chapter 13, offers a holistic approach to care. By marrying conventional treatments with alternative approaches, healthcare can be more comprehensive, addressing multiple facets of patients' health needs. This integration allows practitioners to draw on the strengths of both worlds, potentially reducing the risks associated with any one treatment modality.

In conclusion, managing risks in treatment is a multifaceted process that spans clinical expertise, personalized care, legal compliance, and patient involvement. While alternative treatments like those explored here hold significant promise, the commitment to managing their risks with diligence and transparency can pave the way for safer and more effective healthcare solutions.

Chapter 13: Integrating Traditional and Alternative Medicine

In the ever-evolving landscape of healthcare, the fusion of traditional and alternative medicine offers a promising frontier, yet one fraught with complexity and debate. Navigating this terrain requires an appreciation for the nuanced dynamics at play, from historical precedence to modern-day applications. On one hand, traditional medicine provides a rich tapestry of time-honored practices, deeply rooted in culture and longstanding belief systems. On the other, alternative approaches present a diverse array of innovations and methodologies, often dismissed by skeptics yet embraced by those seeking holistic healing. The challenge lies in bridging these seemingly disparate worlds, forging a collaborative pathway that respects the integrity of both traditions while embracing evidence-based practices. This integration is not merely about merging different treatment modalities but also about fostering a mindset that values open-mindedness, continuous learning, and patient-centered care. Practitioners at the forefront of this integration often find themselves acting as cultural ambassadors, translating therapeutic benefits across disciplines and advocating for systems that honor both science and tradition. As the dialogue between these modalities intensifies, it sparks a broader discourse on the nature of healing itself—inviting medical professionals and health-conscious individuals alike to reconsider what it truly means to be well.

Bridging Two Worlds

As we venture into the realm of integrative medicine, it's vital to understand how traditional and alternative forms of healing intersect. This convergence isn't merely about juxtaposing Western medical practices with ancient approaches like Ayurveda or Traditional Chinese Medicine. It's about crafting a synergistic relationship where both methodologies enhance one another's strengths, leading to better patient outcomes.

The integration of traditional and alternative medicine starts with recognizing the value in each system's perspective. Western medicine is celebrated for its technological advancements and evidence-based approaches. It offers precision and predictability, crucial in acute care scenarios. However, alternative practices often excel in preventive care and maintaining balance in the body, areas where Western medicine sometimes falls short. When we consider diseases that demand long-term management like diabetes or hypertension, alternative therapies can provide supportive measures that improve quality of life.

In some instances, the bridging of these worlds occurs naturally. Consider acupuncture, now an established part of pain management protocols in many U.S. hospitals. Originally viewed with skepticism by Western practitioners, it has gained acceptance through clinical trials demonstrating its efficacy in reducing chronic pain and stress.

Here, tradition complements evidence-based practice, revealing a path forward where collaboration can yield substantial benefits.

Yet, this melding of methodologies doesn't occur in a vacuum. It requires a shift in mindset among healthcare practitioners, many of whom have spent years entrenched in one school of thought. Acceptance and understanding of differing therapeutic approaches demand an open-minded dialogue and a willingness to explore complementarities without bias. For instance, a physician versed in prescribing pharmaceuticals may need to consider how herbal supplements could support a patient's recovery or manage side effects.

Moreover, communication between practitioners from both fields is crucial. Multidisciplinary teams are increasingly common in hospitals and clinics, allowing specialists and holistic healers to discuss best practices tailored to individual patient needs. This collaboration often extends to holistic health coaches, nutritionists, and mental health professionals, cultivating a team-oriented approach that reviews the patient's complete health picture rather than isolated symptoms.

There's a palpable tension, however, in integrating practices that operate on fundamentally different principles. Western medicine typically demands quantifiable results and clinical trial data, while alternative methods may rely on tradition, case studies, or patient testimonials for validation. Bridging this gap involves rigorous research to evaluate the efficacy of alternative treatments, employing scientific methods to assess outcomes in a way that satisfies both perspectives.

Consider, for instance, the practice of using meditation and mindfulness to control anxiety and depression. These techniques, often categorized under alternative medicine, have significant support from scientific studies illustrating changes in brain activity. It demonstrates how alternative practices can be scientifically validated, making them more palatable to traditionally trained clinicians.

Patients also play a fundamental role in bridging these worlds. Today's health-conscious individuals are savvy and often conduct their research, bringing new ideas to their doctors' attention. With access to vast amounts of information online, patients frequently arrive at consultations armed with suggestions for integrative treatments they wish to try. This shift empowers patients but also challenges practitioners to stay informed about a broad spectrum of healing modalities.

We must also acknowledge cultural factors while integrating these worlds. In many societies, alternative medicine systems have profound historical and spiritual significance. For these populations, melding their traditional practices with modern medicine creates a therapeutic model that respects their cultural identity. This cultural sensitivity can enhance patient engagement and compliance, crucial for the success of any treatment regimen.

Finally, legal and regulatory frameworks must evolve to support this integration. As Chapters 10 and 24 suggest, navigating the legal complexities and policy influences can make or break the successful implementation of an integrative approach. Ensuring safe practices while encouraging innovation requires a balanced approach to regulation and an openness to adapt as evidence mounts.

Thus, bridging two worlds in medicine isn't simply a logistical exercise—it's a transformative endeavor that asks more from practitioners and patients alike. It demands a continual evaluation and integration of diverse perspectives, creating a healthcare model that is not only inclusive but also adaptive to the complexities of modern-day health challenges.

Practitioners' Perspectives

The integration of traditional and alternative medicine often presents a unique challenge for practitioners navigating the diverse landscapes of healthcare. On one hand, there's the empirical rigidity of conventional medicine, entrenched in evidence-based practices; on the other, the experiential richness of alternative therapies which, though often lacking in robust clinical validation, provide valuable insights into holistic patient care.

In recent years, the paradigm has gradually shifted, allowing open dialogues between these two worlds. For physicians who once adhered strictly to conventional medicine, the shift represents a significant evolution in how they perceive patient health. Many practitioners now find themselves not only treating symptoms but also considering the broader aspects of wellness, drawing on both traditional knowledge and alternative perspectives.

This shift is not without its complexities. Practitioners often encounter skepticism both from within the medical community and from patients. Traditional training emphasizes diagnosis and treatment rooted in tangible data, but alternative modalities often rely on different approaches — ones that may include the influence of mind-body connections or nutritional interventions featuring unconventional substances like gold and selenium. While such treatments may initially seem fringe, they offer a wealth of anecdotal evidence and historical accounts that cannot be easily dismissed.

Healthcare providers open to integrating alternative practices often describe their experiences as a tapestry woven from diverse threads of healing traditions. One physician noted, "Patients are increasingly knowledgeable and express a desire for treatments that honor their beliefs and experiences." This has fueled a growing interest among practitioners to explore complementary strategies that emphasize patient-centered care.

It's important to realize that while some practitioners view the union of traditional and alternative medicine as an opportunity for innovation, others see it as a contentious issue. Concerns about efficacy, safety, and the potential for unregulated practices to undermine professional standards linger in the minds of many cautious healthcare professionals. These apprehensions underscore the necessity of developing robust guidelines and protocols to safeguard both patients and practitioners.

Successful integration requires a willingness to engage in continuous learning and open-mindedness. Practitioners like Dr. Samuel Greene, a holistic physician, leverage both scientific and traditional knowledge to craft personalized treatment plans. His approach involves engaging patients in conversations about their health histories, needs, and expectations. By doing so, he fosters an environment of trust and collaboration, which he believes is crucial for successful outcomes.

Moreover, many practitioners now advocate for a model of care that is inclusive, recognizing that both modern medicine and traditional healing have valuable contributions. They highlight the need for interdisciplinary teams that can bring together diverse expertise to offer comprehensive care. Integrative clinics, where medical doctors, acupuncturists, nutritionists, and alternative therapists work side by side, are becoming more common, illustrating a practical embodiment of this multidisciplinary approach.

The integration process also sheds light on the importance of informed consent and patient education. Practitioners emphasize that patients must be made aware of the potential benefits and risks of incorporating alternative treatments. This empowers individuals to make informed decisions, aligning with their values and health goals.

Pauline Anders, a nutritionist with a focus on alternative therapies, recounts, "A lot of my work involves demystifying these non-traditional treatments for my patients. By providing them with balanced information, I ensure that they feel supported in their healthcare journey." Her viewpoint reflects a growing trend among practitioners who take on the role of educators as much as caregivers.

Despite the challenges, it's undeniable that practitioners' perspectives on integrating traditional and alternative medicine are evolving, driven by a combination of patient demand, emerging research, and a renewed appreciation for holistic health. This movement encourages a dynamic dialogue within the healthcare community, ultimately aiming to enrich patient care and expand the horizons of modern medicine.

In conclusion, practitioners embracing integrative health models often find themselves at the intersection of tradition and innovation. By valuing scientific rigor and the wisdom of alternative medicine, they contribute to a more inclusive and flexible health system that benefits not just individual patients, but broader society. As this field continues to grow, the perspectives and experiences of these practitioners will play a pivotal role in shaping the future of healthcare.

Chapter 14: Nutritional Aspects of Health

Navigating the complexities of nutrition in our pursuit of health, we quickly discover its pivotal role that stretches beyond mere sustenance. The intersection of diet and alternative treatments, particularly the incorporation of elements like gold and selenium, provokes a rethinking of how we traditionally view nourishment. This chapter embarks on an exploration of not just the basics of dietary contributions to health but also the nuanced impact of targeted supplementation. It's essential to recognize how these elements, within the context of a balanced dietary regimen, might unravel new pathways in disease treatment and prevention. While mainstream nutrition preaches the virtues of vitamins and minerals, delving into the particulars of how such unique trace elements synergize with bodily processes is crucial. The dialogue between conventional dietary guidelines and innovative nutritional strategies highlights an evolving landscape, one where well-informed decisions can potentially transform health outcomes. Unpacking these dynamics, we encourage a thoughtful consideration of nutrition's profound influence on both everyday health and complex medical conditions.

Diet's Role in Treatment

In the intricate web of health, diet stands as a cornerstone of treatment. It's not merely about sustenance—it's a potent tool in the therapeutic arsenal. While medications and therapies address symptoms and underlying conditions, diet can play a crucial role in amplifying these treatments, improving outcomes, and enhancing quality of life.

Understanding how diet integrates into treatment begins with recognizing its foundational impact on the body. Nutrients fuel cellular processes, support immune functions, and aid in the repair and regeneration of tissues. An individual's nutritional status can directly influence their response to treatment and their overall health trajectory. Therefore, when considering treatment strategies, it's imperative to evaluate dietary habits as a complementary intervention.

Particularly in the realm of chronic diseases, diet can transform the treatment landscape. For example, in managing conditions like diabetes, cardiovascular disease, and autoimmune disorders, dietary modifications often lead to significant improvements. Focusing on whole foods, rich in essential nutrients, can help manage disease symptoms and reduce dependency on medication.

A key aspect of diet's role in treatment is its ability to modulate inflammation, a common underpinning in many chronic illnesses.

Diets high in processed foods and sugars are known to exacerbate inflammatory pathways, compromising treatment efficacy. Conversely, anti-inflammatory diets rich in fruits, vegetables, omega-3 fatty acids, and spices such as turmeric can support healing and improve treatment outcomes. It's a simple switch, yet its impacts on health and recovery are profound.

Moreover, an individualized diet plan can cater to specific treatment-related needs. For patients undergoing chemotherapy, maintaining nutrient-dense and easily digestible foods can mitigate treatment side effects like nausea and fatigue. These adjustments not only enhance the treatment experience but can also improve adherence to the therapeutic regimen.

Protein intake plays a significant role, especially in recovery and rehabilitation phases post-treatment. Proteins are vital for muscle repair and maintaining a robust immune system, both of which are critical during treatment recovery. Ensuring adequate protein intake, tailored to the individual's condition and treatment plan, can expedite recovery and reinforce treatment efficacy.

Furthermore, the gut microbiome, though often overlooked, is a significant player in this equation. The balance of gut bacteria, influenced by diet, impacts the immune system and inflammation, as well as the body's ability to metabolize certain medications. A diet rich in probiotics and prebiotics can maintain or restore a healthy gut microbiota, thereby supporting the body's resilience during treatment.

It's important to recognize that diet is not a one-size-fits-all solution in treatments; it must be personalized. Nutrigenomics, the study of how genes interact with diet, is an emerging field that promises tailored dietary interventions based on individual genetic profiles. This approach could revolutionize how nutrition is utilized in treating diseases, making dietary interventions as personalized as the treatments themselves.

The psychological benefits of integrating diet into treatment shouldn't be underestimated. A well-structured diet plan can empower patients, giving them a sense of control over their health journey. This empowerment can translate into improved mental well-being, which is closely linked to treatment success and overall health. The act of making informed dietary choices encourages a proactive attitude towards health, fostering resilience against the challenges of illness and treatment.

In clinical practice, the integration of diet into a treatment plan requires collaboration between healthcare providers, dietitians, and patients. Medical professionals must be equipped with knowledge on how to personalize dietary advice aligned with medical treatments. Dietitians, working alongside doctors, can provide tailored recommendations that harmonize with medical interventions, ensuring that dietary changes complement rather than conflict with prescribed treatments.

It is also worth exploring traditional and cultural dietary practices that may offer insights into treatment methods. Many cultures have long histories of using diet for healing, and modern science continues to uncover the validity and mechanisms behind these practices. Incorporating these holistic perspectives can enrich treatment plans and honor the diverse backgrounds of patients.

The strategic integration of diet in treatment plans is indeed pivotal. As we continue to uncover the complex interplay between diet and health, we must advocate for increased awareness and integration of nutritional strategies within clinical settings. Forward-thinking healthcare systems can leverage dietary interventions, not as an afterthought, but as a fundamental component of therapeutic protocols.

Ultimately, the role of diet in treatment transcends traditional views of nutrition. It is an adaptable, evolving strategy that offers immense potential to enhance health outcomes. By treating diet as a central pillar in treatment planning, we pave the way for holistic care approaches that honor the interconnectedness of body, mind, and nutrition. This shift not only influences individual health trajectories but also embodies a forward-thinking perspective on treatment modalities in the ever-evolving landscape of medicine.

Supplementation with Gold and Selenium

In the realm of alternative medicine, there's a growing intrigue about the potential health benefits of supplementing with gold and selenium. As more people turn to holistic approaches for their health, the intersection of these two elements in nutritional supplementation has generated both excitement and skepticism. Understanding the potential benefits and limitations of such supplementation requires a closer examination of the existing scientific literature, anecdotal evidence, and ongoing research.

Gold, long revered for its symbolic and monetary value, has been associated with health benefits that date back to ancient civilizations. In recent years, interest in its dietary application has increased, especially in forms like monoatomic gold, which purportedly offers enhanced biological availability. Advocates claim that supplementing with gold can enhance cognitive function, support immune health, and improve mental clarity. However, these claims require rigorous scientific evaluation to distinguish fact from speculation.

On the other hand, selenium is a well-recognized essential micronutrient critical for various physiological processes. It's known for its role in antioxidant defense, thyroid hormone metabolism, and immune function. Selenium's potential protective effects against cancer and its importance in mitigating oxidative stress have been extensively studied. While the human body requires selenium in trace amounts, balancing the optimal dose is crucial, as both deficiency and excess intake pose health risks.

Combining these elements in supplementation regimens raises important questions. How do the individual benefits of gold and selenium translate into a synergistic effect when taken together? Currently, scientific understanding of their interaction at a biochemical level is still developing. Preliminary studies hint at promising outcomes, particularly in enhancing antioxidant pathways and improving cellular resilience, but more extensive clinical trials are necessary to substantiate these findings.

A significant concern among medical professionals is the regulation of these supplements. Unlike pharmaceutical drugs, dietary supplements are often subject to less stringent oversight, raising questions about quality control, purity, and accurate labeling. The supplement industry must address these issues to ensure the safety and efficacy of products containing gold and selenium.

The appeal of gold and selenium supplementation lies in the broader narrative of seeking novel solutions to enhance health and prevent disease. Yet, it's critical to ground expectations in evidence-based practice. The scientific community must prioritize well-designed studies that explore not only the potential benefits but also the possible adverse effects and contraindications of such supplementation, particularly in individuals with pre-existing health conditions.

For health-conscious individuals considering gold and selenium supplements, the decision should be informed by a comprehensive understanding of potential health benefits and risks. Consulting with healthcare professionals and relying on products that meet established standards can help individuals make more informed choices about their health practices.

Moving forward, the challenge and opportunity lie in bridging the gap between enthusiasm for novel supplements and the slow but necessary process of scientific validation. This involves encouraging collaboration between researchers, clinicians, and regulatory bodies to advance knowledge and ensure that supplementation practices both reflect sound science and foster genuine health benefits.

Ultimately, the role of supplementation with gold and selenium in the nutritional landscape will be determined by a steady accumulation of high-quality research and a commitment to consumer education. While the mystique surrounding these elements is compelling, only time and continued investigation will reveal their true place in the pantheon of health-promoting strategies.

Chapter 15: Mental and Emotional Dimensions of Healing

The mental and emotional dimensions of healing, though often overshadowed by the physical aspects, play a critical role in the holistic recovery of patients. The profound connection between mind and body suggests that our thoughts and feelings can significantly impact our physical health. By exploring this link, we uncover the psychological benefits explicit in embracing a healing mindset. Techniques such as mindfulness, meditation, and positive visualization aren't just buzzwords; they're evidence-based practices revealing immense potential in the healing journey. Patients often find that addressing emotional well-being alongside traditional medical treatments results in more comprehensive care and enhanced resilience. By integrating these dimensions into a cohesive treatment strategy, health-conscious individuals and medical professionals alike can push the boundaries of recovery, unlocking a more profound understanding of the body's innate capacity for healing. This approach not only fosters a more compassionate understanding of patient care but also opens up new avenues for research and development in alternative medicine. The future of healing lies as much in the capacities of the mind and spirit as it does in the tangible resources of medical science.

Exploring the Mind-Body Connection

Understanding the intricate connection between the mind and body has fascinated scholars and practitioners for centuries. It's an area where science is increasingly recognizing what ancient traditions have long suggested: the state of our minds can significantly influence our physical health. This interplay is at the core of many alternative medicine practices and becomes especially relevant when considering the mental and emotional dimensions of healing. The idea is not merely theoretical—real-world applications and research continue to demonstrate this potent link.

The holistic view of health, where mental and physical components are inseparable, suggests that our emotions and thoughts can manifest in bodily conditions. Stress, for instance, isn't just an emotional burden—it can be a catalyst for diseases. Chronic stress can activate inflammatory pathways in the body, weaken the immune system, and lead to conditions like heart disease and diabetes. On the flip side, positive mental states, such as happiness and tranquility, have been associated with improved immune function and longevity. The evidence is compelling and pushes us to consider new paradigms in health and treatment.

This mind-body connection extends into the realm of mental practices affecting physical outcomes. Techniques like meditation, yoga, and tai chi, rooted in Eastern philosophies, have gained attention in Western medicine for their benefits in alleviating stress and improving overall well-being. The mechanism appears to be through the reduction of cortisol and the enhancement of the parasympathetic nervous system—the body's natural relaxation response. Not only do these practices help calm the mind, but they also rejuvenate the body, presenting a comprehensive approach to health.

Research in psychoneuroimmunology—an interdisciplinary field that studies the interaction between psychological processes and the nervous and immune systems—provides a scientific basis for the mind-body connection. Studies have shown that negative emotions and psychological stress can suppress the immune response, while positive emotions can bolster it, underscoring the physical embodiment of our mental states. This growing research field continues to highlight the necessity of including mental health as a significant component of physical health treatment plans.

Let's not overlook the placebo effect, a classic example illustrating the mind's powerful influence on the body. When patients believe they are receiving treatment, even if it's a sugar pill, they can experience real changes in their condition. This phenomenon isn't merely psychological but involves actual physiological changes in the brain and body. While often discounted in serious medical discussions, the placebo effect is a testament to the power of belief and expectation in healing processes.

The implications of the mind-body connection are profound, offering potential paths for treatment and healing without reliance solely on pharmaceutical interventions. Techniques that promote mental well-being could become vital components of treatment plans, used alongside traditional approaches to address not just symptoms but the underlying emotional states contributing to illness. This integrated approach could lead to more sustainable health outcomes by tackling disease from multiple angles.

However, integrating mind-body practices into conventional medicine isn't without its challenges. The scientific community often requires rigorous evidence, yet not all mind-body interventions can be evaluated through traditional clinical trial methodologies. Despite this, the integration of practices like mindfulness-based stress reduction (MBSR) in diverse medical settings, including oncology and chronic pain management, indicates a growing acceptance. This shift signifies the beginning of a broader appreciation for holistic health methodologies.

Ultimately, exploring the mind-body connection demands a change in how we perceive health—viewing it not as the mere absence of disease but as the attainment of mental and physical harmony. This perspective encourages a more personalized approach to healthcare, recognizing that each individual's mental and emotional state plays a crucial role in their health journey. Adopting such a paradigm could lead to more personalized and effective treatments, enhancing patient care and outcomes.

As we continue to explore and validate the intricate dynamics between mind and body, the potential for transformative healthcare solutions increases. This connection invites healthcare practitioners to be open-minded, innovative, and compassionate, aiming for treatments that are not just about alleviating physical symptoms but also prioritizing mental and emotional well-being. The mind-body connection, once merely philosophical, is now carving out its place in modern medicine with promising possibilities that could redefine our understanding of healing.

Psychological Benefits

The journey of healing is not just a physical endeavor; it's a profound mental and emotional exploration. Tapping into the psychological benefits of alternative treatments like gold and selenium opens up a fascinating world that speaks to our intrinsic need for holistic well-being. This area merges science with the subtle intricacies of human psychology, challenging conventional wisdom and offering a fresh perspective on what it means to heal in mind and body.

Many of us question what makes a treatment effective. Is it purely the biochemistry, or does belief play a role? Psychological benefits, although intangible, are undeniably powerful. They offer comfort, instill hope, and can even catalyze physical healing. When individuals feel a sense of control over their treatment choices, it enhances their emotional resilience. The practice of engaging with alternative medicine facilitates this empowerment, fostering a proactive approach to personal health.

One key aspect is the mind-body connection, which suggests that our thoughts and emotions significantly influence our physical health. This connection becomes particularly evident when exploring how belief and perception impact healing. Expectations can shape results, often referred to as the placebo effect, but perhaps more accurately described as the mental catalyst effect. It's not mere trickery; it's the mind's remarkable ability to manifest physical change. Reports from patients engaging in alternative treatments often cite increased optimism and reduced anxiety, contributing to an improved quality of life.

Imagine a patient diagnosed with a chronic illness. They may feel trapped by their diagnosis, overwhelmed with fear. Introducing an alternative treatment empowers them. It offers a narrative that diverges from despair, promoting a sense of exploration and novelty. This change in perspective can be a potent antidote to the emotional distress that accompanies physical ailments.

Moreover, the communal aspect of alternative medicine can't be overlooked. Joining communities of like-minded individuals who are exploring similar paths can boost morale and provide emotional support. The shared experiences and discussions contribute to a sense of belonging and understanding, elements crucial for emotional well-being. Patients feel less isolated in their journeys, discovering solace in shared experiences and wisdom.

Emotional resilience, or the ability to navigate through emotional challenges healthily, is another psychological benefit of incorporating these elements into one's healing strategy. Interaction with alternative medicine can instill a sense of hope, which cultivates resilience. The belief in the possibility of recovery can drive individuals to persevere, even in the face of daunting medical challenges. It's about adopting a mindset that doesn't solely focus on curing but also on thriving despite the circumstances.

Cultural narratives and historical usage of gold and selenium add another layer to their psychological appeal. Many cultures have cherished these elements as sacred, attributing them with mystical healing properties. This historical reverence impacts the modern psyche, making the use of such treatments feel like an alignment with ancient wisdom. Such alignment can offer a sense of peace and tradition, grounding individuals in their healing journey.

Critics might argue that focusing on psychological benefits is akin to grasping at straws when tangible results are lacking. However, it's essential to recognize that these benefits do not operate in isolation. They accompany physical changes, potentially enhancing the efficacy of treatments. As alternative treatments continue to gain attention, their psychological impact becomes a crucial component of the discussion, one that bridges the gap between pure science and human experience.

This integration of psychological benefits doesn't aim to replace conventional treatments but rather to complement them. The dual approach addresses both the measurable and immeasurable aspects of healing. By bridging the divide between the scientific and emotional spheres, we open ourselves to a more nuanced understanding of health. Here lies an opportunity for medical professionals to incorporate a holistic approach that honors both the technical and introspective realms of healing.

In conclusion, the psychological benefits associated with alternative treatments like gold and selenium are multi-faceted, deeply tied to our perception and experience of health. They offer a holistic dimension to healing, emphasizing the importance of mental well-being alongside physical health. This approach advocates for a balance that respects the complexities of human nature, positioning psychology as a powerful ally in the art and science of healing.

Chapter 16: Testimonials from Medical Professionals

In the heart of modern medicine, where evidence and efficacy reign supreme, a growing number of physicians find themselves captivated by the potential of alternative treatments like monoatomic gold and selenium. These medical professionals, many of whom once viewed such treatments with skepticism, now recount tales from the frontlines where traditional practices meet innovative solutions. Their testimonials don't merely echo hope but underline tangible outcomes observed in their patients, mingling anecdotal evidence with clinical observations. Such narratives provide a bridge between established practices and emerging modalities, urging the broader medical community to reconsider the rigid boundaries that often separate alternative and conventional medicine. This chapter highlights their stories, exploring how these professionals reconcile their rigorous training with the emerging possibilities of alternative treatments, thereby fostering a nuanced dialogue within clinical environments. Whether through pioneering discussions at conferences or quietly implementing changes in their practices, these doctors are not just witnesses but active participants in a medical evolution, advocating for an integrated approach to patient care that harmonizes science and innovation.

Doctors on the Frontlines

The relationship between doctors and alternative medicine has always been a complex one. Yet, it's undeniable that some medical professionals are pioneering a thoughtful integration of alternative treatments into conventional practices. In a world where traditional and alternative health paradigms often collide, these doctors stand at the interface, navigating a landscape filled with skepticism, hope, and evidence-based practice.

On the frontlines of healthcare, doctors confront the daily realities of human suffering. It's no wonder that many of them seek more effective solutions, sometimes turning to unconventional methods like the use of monoatomic gold and selenium. This isn't simply about adopting new trends; it's about finding ways to enhance patient care outcomes, especially when traditional methods fall short. Their journey is filled with challenges and breakthroughs, where scientific rigor meets open-minded experimentation.

The quest for integration, while exciting, comes with ethical and practical challenges. Balancing evidence-based medicine with personal patient experience requires a nuanced approach. For doctors like Jason Kim, a general practitioner working in rural clinics, this often means weighing the lack of comprehensive clinical data against real-world patient feedback. According to Kim, the key is not just in the treatment itself but in crafting an open dialogue with patients. He believes educating them about both the potential benefits and

Despite these success stories, doctors on the frontlines often face criticism from peers who caution against straying from tested methods. The tension arises from differing interpretations of what constitutes 'valid' evidence. Some strictly adhere to the gold standard of randomized controlled trials, while others argue for a more flexible understanding, one that includes patient narratives and smaller observational studies. This debate is seen in conferences and research circles, shaping the future of medical practices globally.

The divide between alternative and conventional medicine may not close overnight, but the work of these forward-thinking doctors is a step toward a more integrated healthcare ecosystem. Not only do they provide immediate patient benefits, but they also contribute to a growing body of knowledge that future medical research can build upon. Docs on the field see first-hand the limitations of dogmatic thinking and the possibilities when a multi-faceted approach to health is embraced.

As these doctors continue to document and publish their findings, their impact extends beyond immediate patient care. They influence policy makers, healthcare organizations, and insurance companies to consider and sometimes adopt alternative methods. The path is fraught with obstacles, but their determination fuels a trickle-down effect that could see more widespread acceptance and integration of alternative options in mainstream medicine.

Summing up, doctors on the frontlines represent a vital intersection in current medical practice. Their willingness to explore, validate, and sometimes challenge the status quo is paving the way for a more inclusive definition of healthcare. They teach us that medicine's ultimate goal remains, as ever, to heal and to give hope—to explore every avenue that might lead to healthier lives. As we bridge the gap between theory and practice, these pioneering doctors remind us that vigilance, open-mindedness, and compassion are, and must remain, the cornerstones of medical practice.

Bridging Clinical Practices

In the evolving landscape of medicine, bridging the divide between conventional and alternative approaches is becoming increasingly necessary. Medical professionals are at the forefront of this integration, acting as conduits between traditional medical protocols and innovative, holistic treatments. Their unique vantage point allows them to glean insights from both sides, creating a hybrid approach that can offer deeper insights into patient care.

One of the most discussed topics among medical professionals today is the incorporation of alternative treatments like monoatomic gold and selenium, which have historical roots but are finding renewed interest in modern practice. In clinical settings, doctors are seeing an increasing number of patients who either inquire about or are already supplementing with these elements. This trend forces professionals to critically assess such treatments, weighing anecdotal benefits against scientific validation.

Integrating practices isn't just about accepting new treatments but involves a paradigm shift in thinking. Physicians and health practitioners are now compelled to go beyond the confines of classical medical texts, delving into a variety of sources, including naturopathy and ancient alchemical practices. These modalities, once relegated to the fringes of healthcare, are seeing a resurgence as both patients and practitioners seek more personalized healthcare solutions.

At the heart of this integration is the need for a multidisciplinary approach. Specialists in oncology, nutrition, and psychology, among others, are collaborating more openly to explore how alternative practices can complement conventional treatment. For example, in oncology, there's emerging discourse on monoatomic gold's potential synergistic effects when combined with traditional cancer therapies. While clinical trials are in their nascent stages, anecdotal evidence shared by informed practitioners can lay the groundwork for more focused scientific inquiries.

Medical professionals are also addressing the skepticism and criticisms that often accompany alternative treatments. Bridging clinical practices mandates an open dialogue between skeptics and proponents. Doctors, who are traditionally trained to trust in peer-reviewed, double-blind studies, are now tasked with reconciling these scientific methods with anecdotal evidence that doesn't always fit neatly into established protocols.

Despite the challenges, there has been a positive shift toward viewing patient testimonials and alternative treatments not as contradictions to modern medicine, but as complements. This doesn't undermine the need for caution and critical evaluation; instead, it highlights the potential for these approaches to coexist. Medical professionals aim to harness the best of both worlds to provide patients with options tailored to their unique conditions and preferences.

The shift is more than philosophical; it has practical implications. Medical conferences and symposiums are gradually beginning to include sessions on alternative treatments, eliciting a blend of curiosity and cautious optimism. This inclusion allows professionals to exchange ideas, scrutinize emerging data, and share their clinical experiences, fostering a collective understanding that's crucial for informed decision-making.

In attempting to bridge these practices, one enduring challenge remains: the regulation of alternative treatments. Without a standardized framework, medical professionals often tread a tricky path, navigating both legal and ethical minefields. Here, their testimonials are pivotal, serving as critical commentary on the efficacy and safety of alternative approaches. Their voices can shape guidelines that balance innovation with patient safety.

As more professionals become vocal about these integrations, there's a growing recognition of the importance of patient education. Practitioners are not just healthcare providers but educators, tasked with demystifying alternative treatments for their patients. They provide a measured perspective that helps patients make informed decisions, bridging the knowledge gap that often exists between scientific literature and lay understanding.

In summary, bridging clinical practices is an exciting, albeit complex, undertaking. It demands medical professionals to be not only knowledgeably adaptive but also champions of collaborative care. The tapestry of modern medicine is richly woven with threads from both established and emerging practices, each contributing to a nuanced approach to health and healing. This integration represents a shift towards a more patient-centric model, where the ultimate goal is a universally accessible, evidence-informed healthcare system. By fostering collaboration among medical professionals, the potential exists to truly revolutionize patient care, closing the gap between diverse medical ideologies and establishing a seamless continuity in treatment methods.

Chapter 17: The Future of Gold and Selenium in Medicine

The trajectory of gold and selenium in medicine hints at an exciting intersection between ancient wisdom and modern innovation. As emerging research continues to push boundaries, these elements show promise for broader acceptance in mainstream medical treatments. Scientists are exploring their synergistic potential, revealing biochemical interactions that could revolutionize therapies for chronic conditions, potentially enhancing recovery rates and improving quality of life. Yet, the challenge lies in navigating the blurred lines between alternative and conventional methods. Researchers are driven by a need to substantiate claims with robust evidence while ensuring patient safety. This burgeoning field beckons innovation, urging us to reconsider preconceived notions about medicinal solutions. The future will likely see gold and selenium embedded in personalized treatment paradigms, as scientific rigor and open-minded exploration open new therapeutic frontiers.

Emerging Research Directions

The intersection of gold and selenium in medicine is an intriguing frontier, one that pushes the boundaries of traditional scientific inquiry. Recent studies have shifted focus toward uncovering the potent synergistic effects these elements might have. This emerging research is transforming initial skepticism into a cautiously optimistic examination of gold and selenium as potential game-changers in health and medicine.

Groundbreaking research is currently underway in esteemed universities and private labs around the globe to explore how gold nanoparticles can be engineered to target cancer cells with unprecedented precision. These tiny particles promise to revolutionize treatment methodologies, offering a targeted approach that minimizes damage to surrounding healthy cells. What's captivating about this line of inquiry is not just its scientific novelty, but its implications for improving patient outcomes considerably and with fewer side effects.

Another compelling avenue of research involves selenium's role as an antioxidant. Numerous studies are examining its potential in reducing oxidative stress – a primary contributor to chronic diseases. This entails a complex dance between selenium's normal biological functions and its role as a therapeutic agent. By focusing on its ability to bolster the body's immune response, researchers hope to unlock selenium's broader therapeutic potential.

The scientific community has also begun exploring the combination of gold and selenium in combatting neurological disorders. Gold's conductivity and the neuroprotective qualities of selenium hint at a collaborative dynamic which may offer new treatment pathways for diseases like Alzheimer's and Parkinson's. These early investigations suggest that these metallic elements can play a critical role in neural tissue regeneration, paving the way for treatments that could potentially reverse or halt the progression of neurodegenerative diseases.

One of the more promising aspects of research into gold and selenium lies in personalized medicine. Scientists are working diligently to understand how genetic variations influence an individual's response to these treatments. By tailoring interventions to an individual's genetic makeup, medical professionals can potentially increase efficacy while minimizing risks. The future might see treatment plans that use gold and selenium not as standalone therapies but as integral components of a highly personalized and multi-faceted approach.

In parallel, there's an increasing focus on understanding how these elements influence cell signaling pathways. A deeper knowledge of how gold and selenium interact with cellular processes is crucial. Scientists are mapping out these intricate pathways to better inform how these metals can be harnessed to influence biological functions favorably. This includes measuring how selenium supplementation affects metabolic pathways and how gold can alter protein interactions within the body.

While much of this research is in preliminary phases, the implications are far-reaching. There's an enthusiastic drive among researchers to explore these unknown territories. With advancements in nanotechnology, the ability to manipulate gold at an atomic level provides exciting possibilities for future breakthroughs. The subtle biochemical nuances of selenium, too, are being dissected with increasing focus, anticipation, and a fair amount of scientific rigor.

Moreover, collaborative international efforts are underway to share findings and enhance the global understanding of these metals in medicine. Conferences and symposia are becoming platforms for discussing trials and errors, epitomizing the scientific principle of learning through repetition and collaboration. Shared databases and cross-border research initiatives further compound the growing body of knowledge, incrementally contributing to a comprehensive exploration of gold and selenium's medical potential.

Looming large on the horizon is the potential for these elements to become integral to mainstream medicine. As clinical trials expand and findings accumulate, regulatory bodies may start to recognize these treatments' efficacy as evidenced-based. This would require not only deep investigations but also pragmatic considerations of how these treatments can be standardized for public use.

Financial investments are also crucial to advancing this research. Grants and funding from both public institutions and private entities are essential for sustaining long-term projects. The economic potential of breakthroughs in using gold and selenium for medical purposes could benefit both citizens and economies if managed thoughtfully and ethically.

Questions remain, of course, and not all research will yield the desired results. However, it is this relentless pursuit of understanding – a characteristic so deeply ingrained in scientific inquiry – that propels these research directions forward. What is emerging is a landscape rich with possibility, a tapestry woven with curiosity, ambition, and the hope for medical revolutions that once seemed a flight of fancy.

Potential for Mainstream Adoption

As the world of medicine continually evolves, the potential for integrating gold and selenium into mainstream healthcare grows more intriguing. Potential catalysts for this adoption include successful clinical trials, emerging research that illuminates their mechanisms of action, and growing anecdotal evidence from patients and professionals alike. But the journey to mainstream acceptance isn't straightforward. The medical community's cautious approach to adopting new treatments is deeply rooted in scientific rigor and patient safety.

One of the primary factors fueling interest in gold and selenium is their appeal as alternative treatments. As healthcare costs soar and chronic diseases become more prevalent, patients and practitioners seek additional tools to improve outcomes. Gold, with its history dating back to ancient alchemy, and selenium, revered for its antioxidant properties, present compelling narratives that blend both Eastern and Western medicinal philosophies.

This blend is crucial. Modern-day medicine doesn't operate in isolation. The integration of gold and selenium would require a multifaceted approach, balancing ancient wisdom with contemporary science. Out of necessity, healthcare practitioners are consistently looking to broaden their treatment paradigms, especially when traditional approaches fail to yield expected results.

It's within this gap that gold and selenium may find fertile ground for acceptance.

One of the hurdles to their mainstream adoption is the inherent skepticism from the scientific community. Gold and selenium, often labeled under the umbrella of "alternative treatments," must undergo rigorous scientific validation to dispel notions of pseudoscience. This isn't just a battle for credibility; it's a crucial step in ensuring patient safety and efficacy. Given the complex biochemistry and potential interactions involved, understanding these elements' exact mechanisms is paramount.

The process is underway. Studies are increasingly focusing on gold and selenium's combined effects, examining their synergistic potential. This area of exploration is fascinating because it taps into the body's natural pathways, potentially offering new ways to enhance traditional treatments. As research methodologies improve and tools become more sophisticated, the understanding of these elements' roles in the body deepens, offering tantalizing possibilities.

Beyond the scientific sphere, public perception plays a critical role in the adoption of new treatments. Media coverage and education campaigns heavily influence this perception. When publicized appropriately, patient success stories and professional testimonials can serve as powerful motivators, helping to bridge the gap between skepticism and acceptance. The role of advocacy groups can't be downplayed, either, as they often propel these narratives to the forefront of public consciousness.

Furthermore, the ethical considerations surrounding the use of alternative treatments can't be ignored. As these treatments gain traction, a delicate balance must be struck between offering hope and ensuring treatments are grounded in reality. Ethical dilemmas, such as consent and transparency, must be vigilantly managed to preserve trust between patients and healthcare providers.

Legal frameworks also significantly impact potential adoption. With regulatory hurdles inherently tied to new treatments, navigating these complexities is crucial. Governments and health organizations worldwide are tasked with evaluating emerging treatments for safety and efficacy. Establishing clear legal pathways for approval not only accelerates adoption but also reinforces the treatments' legitimacy.

There's also the question of accessibility. For gold and selenium to be truly mainstream, ensuring they are available across diverse socioeconomic landscapes is essential. This involves collaborating with insurance companies, policymakers, and healthcare providers to create feasible payment models and protocols that don't disadvantage anyone.

Given the current trajectory of healthcare evolution, the rise of personalized medicine offers a promising angle. Techniques like genetic profiling are revolutionizing how treatments are tailored to individuals, enhancing both effectiveness and safety. Gold and selenium could play a pivotal role here, providing customizable treatments that align with patients' unique physiological needs.

Looking towards the future, the integration of technology in medicine further supports the potential for these treatments to go mainstream. From advanced diagnostic tools to machine learning algorithms, tech innovations are reshaping research methods and treatment protocols. Such advancements could expedite the findings that are so essential for establishing gold and selenium in mainstream medicine.

Finally, the intersection of global perspectives cannot be overstated. Different cultures have unique approaches to health and healing, and embracing these diverse perspectives can foster broader acceptance. As gold and selenium are studied and utilized in varying cultural contexts, international case studies could illuminate valuable insights, supporting global integration.

The adoption of gold and selenium in mainstream medicine represents a confluence of history, science, culture, and ethics. While challenges exist, the ongoing dialogue between conventional and alternative practitioners suggests a fertile ground for collaboration. The potential is vast, and the journey to mainstream adoption, while complex, holds promise for the future of medicine.

Chapter 18: Building Awareness and Education

Educating the public about alternative medicine revolves around bridging the gap between scientific nuance and everyday understanding. To tackle this challenge, we must dive deep into how information can be both a catalyst for empowerment and a cornerstone for change. While unraveling the layers of public perception, it's crucial to recognize the roles played by media narratives, cultural beliefs, and personal testimonies in shaping attitudes. Awareness campaigns must be built on a foundation of transparent information, leaning heavily on the credibility of medical professionals and validated research. By harnessing persuasive communication strategies, advocates can foster a more informed public that's equipped to make health-conscious decisions. At its core, education isn't just about imparting knowledge; it's about inspiring individuals to think critically and act decisively on their health journeys.

Public Perception and Influence

Public perception plays a pivotal role in the acceptance and advocacy of alternative medicine treatments like those involving monoatomic gold and selenium. While the mainstream medical community often casts a skeptical eye on non-conventional approaches, a growing number of patients and health-conscious individuals are showing interest. This shift in perception can largely be attributed to an increased curiosity about holistic wellness and dissatisfaction with traditional solutions. The public's fascination with alternative medicine is not just a trend—it's a movement driven by both anecdote and evidence.

Media coverage is one of the most powerful influences on public perception. Television shows, documentaries, and online articles highlighting miraculous recoveries or promising scientific studies can sway public opinion significantly. With the rise of social media platforms, where information—fact or fiction—spreads like wildfire, shaping public perception has both broadened and become more challenging. In some cases, sensationalism trumps scientific accuracy, leading to both increased interest and deepened skepticism. The tension between sensational media stories and responsible journalism remains a critical factor in how alternative medicine is perceived.

Moreover, word of mouth and personal testimonials often carry more weight for individuals than impersonal studies. When someone hears a story of a friend's or family member's success with alternative treatments, it personalizes the potential benefits. Such stories are powerful and, in many ways, uncontrollable in their spread. This organic storytelling can create a trusting community bound by shared experiences, but it can also lead to misinformation and unrealistic expectations if not matched with factual guidance.

Economic factors also shape public perception. As healthcare costs rise, many people view alternative medicine as a more affordable option. While initial costs for supplements or alternative therapies might seem lower, the long-term financial implications and efficacy are factors that prospective users must consider. The perception of alternative treatments being cost-effective may not always align with reality, especially if users do not experience the desired outcomes and opt for a return to conventional treatments.

In a society increasingly driven by data, educational initiatives can effectively alter perception by providing clear, factual information about alternative treatments. Educational campaigns focusing on potential benefits, risks, and the science behind treatments can empower individuals to make informed decisions. When respected institutions and professionals endorse or discuss alternative treatments with an open mind, it can lend credibility and weight to public opinion, leading to a more informed and balanced view.

Healthcare professionals themselves can significantly influence public perception. When doctors and practitioners openly discuss both the possibilities and limitations of alternative treatments without dismissing them outright, it can transform patient attitudes. Integrative medicine practices, which adopt both traditional and alternative methods, can serve as powerful examples for successfully bridging the gap in public confidence. Patients tend to trust practitioners who acknowledge all potential treatment paths, thus aligning medical guidance with personal health goals.

Controversies and myths surrounding alternative treatments also play into public perception, often leading to polarized views. While skepticism is healthy, outright dismissal without consideration stifles exploration and innovation. Key to this dynamic is how the public processes information. The challenge lies in striking a balance between a cautious, evidence-based approach and maintaining the openness necessary for exploring new possibilities. Effective communication strategies that promote critical thinking without discouraging inquiry are paramount.

Professional organizations and advocacy groups can facilitate informed perceptions by often engaging in public discourse, setting standards, and guiding consumer understanding. Advocacy can take many forms, from policy lobbying to grassroots education campaigns. When these groups effectively communicate the complexities surrounding alternative medicine, they help build a more nuanced appreciation across diverse audience segments, from the curious layperson to the staunch skeptic.

Remember, public perception is not static—it evolves as new information emerges and public attitudes shift. In many ways, the journey of integrating alternative treatments into accepted medical practice parallels the broader societal trend towards personalized and preventive approaches to health. In recent years, recognition of the mind-body connection and the impact of lifestyle on health has only reinforced this trend, signaling significant shifts on the horizon for alternative medicine.

Ultimately, the intersection of personal belief systems, cultural influences, and scientific inquiry forms the basis of public perception in alternative medicine. As narratives grow richer and more diverse, the discussion around these treatments becomes a complex tapestry of hope, evidence, skepticism, and acceptance. As these dialogues continue to grow, they offer a fertile ground for advancing both scientific understanding and societal acceptance, forming a crucial part of the evolving landscape of healthcare.

Strategies for Advocacy

Creating awareness and building education around health solutions, particularly those in alternative medicine, requires well-considered advocacy strategies. The complex, often controversial, nature of treatments like monoatomic gold and selenium emphasizes the need for targeted approaches. To shift perceptions and foster understanding, advocates must employ a multifaceted strategy that taps into emotional narratives, scientific evidence, and public discourse.

Advocacy strategies rooted in storytelling can profoundly impact how these alternative treatments are perceived by health-conscious individuals and medical professionals alike. Real-life stories of recovery and hope can humanize what is often seen as an abstract, scientific discussion. This narrative approach doesn't just present an idea but goes deeper by illustrating the tangible effects on human lives. Effective advocates harness these testimonials to build emotional resonance, creating a connection that numbers and data alone can't achieve.

While narratives are powerful, they must be grounded in credible, scientific evidence to gain the trust of a skeptical audience. Detailed case studies and peer-reviewed clinical trials should be core components of any advocacy effort, as they offer verifiable proof of efficacy and safety. This dual approach—emotion tempered by logic—helps to bridge the gap between empirical evidence and personal beliefs.

Engaging in public discourse is another critical element. Holding seminars, webinars, and workshops can stimulate discussion and dispel myths surrounding alternative treatments. By creating platforms for open dialogue, advocates can address misconceptions directly and encourage critical examination rather than blind acceptance or dismissal. These initiatives should aim at sparking curiosity and prompting individuals to explore new perspectives on health and wellness.

Sustainability of advocacy efforts often hinges upon collaboration and coalition-building. Bringing together diverse groups of stakeholders—including health professionals, researchers, and patient organizations—strengthens the voice of advocacy and broadens its reach. Such alliances can create a more extensive and influential network, amplifying the advocacy message far beyond what any single entity might achieve alone.

Social media's impact on information dissemination in today's digital age cannot be overstated. Platforms like Twitter, Instagram, and Facebook offer avenues for advocates to reach broader audiences rapidly. However, the challenge lies in maintaining message integrity amidst a sea of misinformation. Content must be crafted carefully, balancing engaging headlines with accurate, substantive information. Regular interaction with followers can help keep the dialogue ongoing and vibrant.

In tandem with these efforts, engaging influencers, particularly those with credibility in health and wellness, can significantly enhance advocacy campaigns. When trusted figures endorse a treatment or therapy, it can sway public opinion and motivate personal health explorations. This strategy is particularly effective if the influencer's vision aligns with the core values of the advocacy message.

Advocates should not overlook the role of education in schools and community centers as a fertile ground for sowing seeds of awareness. Introducing educational programs and workshops focused on holistic and alternative health can enact early positive shifts in perception. These initiatives don't just educate the young but also often reach their families, extending the scope of awareness efforts.

Ultimately, successful advocacy is adaptive and responsive, recognizing that what resonates with one group might not with another. Regular feedback from the community and critical analysis of advocacy outcomes are vital in refining strategies. Flexibility, coupled with persistence, ensures that advocacy remains relevant in an ever-evolving landscape of health care and societal attitudes.

Given the controversial nature of alternative treatments, advocates must prepare for resistance, particularly from entities invested in conventional modalities. Effective counter-strategies involve factual rebuttals, maintaining a focus on patient autonomy and choice, and promoting the idea of integrative medicine, where complementary treatments are part of a broader, inclusive health strategy.

As the dialogue on alternative treatments continues to evolve, advocacy serves as both a compass and a vehicle guiding public perception. By tapping into human emotions, backing claims with scientific credibility, and maintaining an adaptive approach, advocates can pave the way for a broader acceptance and understanding of innovative health solutions.

Chapter 19: Developing Safe Dosages and Protocols

Creating safe dosages and protocols is crucial in the integration of alternative medicines like monoatomic gold and selenium into contemporary therapeutic practices. This pursuit requires a delicate balancing act, harnessing the insights of biochemical research and individual variability. By tailoring treatments to individual needs, practitioners aim to maximize efficacy while minimizing risks, yet this personalization raises complex questions of monitoring, patient involvement, and adherence. The development of protocols isn't merely about scaling traditional practices to modern contexts but is an ongoing conversation between history, current scientific understanding, and future innovation. Unlocking the potential of these elements safely demands not only rigorous scientific inquiry but also an ethical commitment to patient welfare and informed consent, a truly multidisciplinary challenge that invites both caution and creativity.

Tailoring Treatments to Individuals

In the contemporary landscape of medicine, the term "personalization" has garnered attention akin to a revolution. No longer is it sufficient to prescribe a standard regimen to every patient; the complexities of human biology demand a nuanced approach. This calls for tailoring treatments to individuals, especially when working with alternative therapies such as gold and selenium—a practice that aims to strike the delicate balance between efficacy and safety.

It begins with understanding the unique biological makeup of each individual. Every person possesses distinct genetic, metabolic, and epigenetic attributes that influence how they respond to treatment. Just as a melody changes with each instrument, individual responses to substances like gold and selenium vary tremendously. Hence, the need to assess genetic markers and metabolic rates prior to initiating any treatment becomes paramount. These assessments can guide practitioners in predicting possible reactions, thereby reducing risks.

Yet, it's not only about genetics; lifestyle factors present another layer of complexity. Dietary habits, environmental exposures, and stress levels intertwine with biology to affect how treatment protocols manifest in individuals. A practitioner aiming to tailor a treatment plan for someone must consider such lifestyle elements. This holistic perspective allows for the creation of a plan that syncs with the patient's daily routine, making adherence more likely and beneficial outcomes more achievable.

Moreover, personal health history is a critical aspect of designing individualized protocols. Previous medical conditions, ongoing treatments, and even family medical history provide insights into what a patient might tolerate or require. For instance, a person with a history of autoimmune conditions may react differently to selenium supplementation compared to someone without such a background. This history-centered approach ensures that treatments are not only personalized but also precisely targeted.

Once all facets of an individual's makeup are understood, the actual process of tailoring begins. This often involves initial trial and error—beginning with minimal dosages and gradually adjusting based on monitoring results. Through regular observation and feedback loops, dosages can be fine-tuned to meet the individual's specific needs. It's a dance of precision; too much or too little could tip the scale away from therapeutic benefits, potentially inducing adverse reactions.

The role of technology cannot be disregarded in this personalization crusade. Advancements in data analytics and wearable health devices are opening doors to real-time monitoring that aids in tailoring treatments. For example, integrating wearable tech can provide continuous data on a patient's response to a treatment regimen, allowing for immediate adjustments. This dynamic interaction forms the crux of truly individualized medicine, where adjustments are based not just on periodic consultations but ongoing data.

Furthermore, this process isn't just about measuring and adjusting—and adjusting again. Communication plays a pivotal role. Practitioners must engage in open dialogues with their patients, ensuring that there is a mutual understanding of the proposed regimen and expectations. Patients should be encouraged to report not just physical but also emotional responses to the treatment. Such feedback enriches the refinement process, ensuring that the treatment aligns with the patient's values and experiences.

Incorporating psychological insights also enriches the treatment plan. By recognizing the emotional and mental state of the patient, practitioners can tweak regimens to include supportive therapies. For example, integrating stress management techniques or mindfulness exercises may enhance the overall efficacy of physical treatments. This multifaceted approach aligns treatment with the broader goal of holistic health, acknowledging the intricate interplay between mind and body.

Tailoring treatments to individuals is, therefore, a multi-dimensional task. It requires a balance of art and science, intuition and data, personalization and standardization. Practitioners must be willing to transcend standard protocols and engage in continuous learning alongside their patients. As each treatment deepens our understanding of how gold and selenium can be optimally utilized, we forge paths toward more effective and personalized strategies, potentially transforming the landscape of not just alternative medicine but healthcare on the whole.

The conversation on individualized treatment continues to evolve, shaped by ongoing research and clinical discoveries. In this realm, the capacity to learn from each patient, to discern patterns, and to adapt accordingly is of unmatched importance. The lessons learned in tailoring these treatments could redefine how medicine is practiced, shifting from a one-size-fits-all paradigm to a more nuanced, individualized approach.

This paradigm shift towards personalized treatment echoes a broader societal trend of seeking individuality in all aspects of life. As the field progresses and methods continue to innovate, it's plausible that personalized protocols will become the norm rather than the exception, benefiting an ever-evolving understanding of human health. The road to fully individualized treatment is complex and requires diligence and compassion, but it's a journey worth undertaking for its potential to improve patient outcomes significantly.

Protocols for Safe Usage

In the realm of alternative medicine, the pursuit of safe and effective dosages is paramount. This is especially true when it comes to using substances like monoatomic gold and selenium, which hold promise but also warrant careful handling. Understanding their potential benefits while minimizing risks requires adhering to well-established protocols. This involves not just specifying the correct dosages, but also understanding the interactions these substances might have with each other and with the human body.

Developing protocols for safe usage begins with a foundation of scientific inquiry. Clinical research plays a crucial role in determining safe thresholds and effective dosages that are tailored to individuals' needs. It's not just about finding a one-size-fits-all solution; personalized medicine has underscored the importance of customization in healthcare. This means considering factors like age, baseline health conditions, genetic predispositions, and even lifestyle when outlining a protocol.

One essential aspect involves understanding the basic pharmacokinetics and pharmacodynamics of these elements. Pharmacokinetics involves how a substance is absorbed, distributed, metabolized, and excreted by the body. In contrast, pharmacodynamics deals with the biochemical and physiological effects, particularly how a substance influences cellular processes.

Knowing both is key to formulating protocols that balance effectiveness with safety.

Effective protocols account for potential interactions, not just with other medications but with dietary factors and lifestyle choices. For instance, the presence of certain foods or supplements can alter how the body absorbs monoatomic elements or selenium, potentially enhancing or diminishing their intended effects. Cross-disciplinary studies often uncover these interactions, helping to refine these protocols further.

However, protocols must also be flexible and adaptive. Medical practitioners should be ready to update them based on emerging research and patient feedback. For instance, anecdotal evidence from patients might reveal unexpected benefits or side effects that require tweaking the prescribed dosage or frequency. This fluid approach helps keep protocols relevant and scientifically grounded.

On a structural level, implementing protocols requires clear communication with patients. Transparency is vital, as is educating patients on what to expect and how to monitor their responses. It's not just about handing over a dosage chart; it's about encouraging patients to report changes in their health, whether positive or negative. Regular follow-ups and open channels for communication make this approach feasible.

The question of dosage can also vary greatly depending on ongoing research, much of which is still underway. For instance, small-scale studies might suggest differing effective amounts compared to larger, more comprehensive trials. This points to the need for continuous adjustment and vigilant attention to the latest scientific insights. Protocols can thus evolve substantially over time, reflecting new understandings and applications.

Moreover, rigorous documentation is an often underscored part of the process. Detailed records of patient responses can provide invaluable data not only for the individual involved but also for broader studies, paving the way for further refinement of protocols. This approach transforms patient care into a collaborative, evidence-driven endeavor.

Ethical considerations also come into play when developing these protocols. It's imperative to weigh the risks against potential benefits responsibly. Patients need to be informed of both, ensuring that consent is both informed and voluntary. This ethical conduct builds trust and credibility within the sphere of alternative treatments.

Finally, disseminating these protocols among healthcare professionals is necessary to ensure consistent and standardized treatment methodologies. Workshops, seminars, and peer-reviewed publications can be effective means to achieve this. By engaging the medical community, it becomes possible to harness collective insights and continuously refine these practices.

In summary, the development of safe usage protocols for monoatomic gold and selenium is a nuanced and dynamic process. It integrates scientific research, ethical considerations, and patient-centered care, requiring flexibility and ongoing adaptation to remain effective. In doing so, it not only promises to enhance treatment outcomes but also elevates the standards for alternative medicine solutions, positioning them more securely within the broader healthcare landscape.

Chapter 20: Global Perspectives on Gold and Selenium

Across the globe, the use of gold and selenium in health practices reflects a rich tapestry of cultural interpretations and applications. In regions like Asia, gold's luxurious aura extends beyond adornment, finding its place in traditional remedies that promise rejuvenation and healing. Contrast this with Western skepticism, where scientific rigor demands empirical evidence, yet curiosity about these elements persists. Meanwhile, in parts of Africa and South America, selenium's role in nutrition and disease prevention captivates researchers seeking solutions tailored to local health challenges. These international narratives underscore a fascinating paradox: while scientific communities strive for consensus on efficacy and safety, cultural stories and individual testimonies project a persistent belief in the transformative power of these elements. As global discourse evolves, the convergence of modern science and traditional wisdom may unveil unprecedented insights into the nuanced relationship between gold, selenium, and human health.

Cultural Views and Practices

Gold and selenium are not merely chemical elements; they are imbued with rich cultural narratives that span continents and millennia. Throughout history, these elements have been revered not just for their material value or biological significance but for their symbolic and spiritual associations. Around the world, varying beliefs and practices have given shape to our understanding of these elements, forming a complex tapestry of tradition and modernity.

In several cultures, gold has been synonymous with the divine and the eternal. The ancient Egyptians considered it the flesh of the gods, a belief that intertwined spiritual reverence with tangible opulence. Temples and tombs glittered with the hues of gold, signifying both earthly power and a conduit to the afterlife. This belief was not isolated; in other ancient cultures from the Incas to the Hindu civilizations, gold was often seen as a celestial gift, embodying purity and enlightenment. Its allure has etched a permanent mark on religious practices, often used in rituals, artifacts, and sacred symbols.

On the other hand, selenium doesn't share the same opulent history as gold. Its cultural footprint is subtler, yet no less fascinating. In certain indigenous communities, the presence of selenium-rich plants has been utilized for its health benefits, unknowingly integrating it into traditional medicine practices. In China, a culture renowned for its ancient healing wisdom, selenium-rich tea blends and herbal regimes reflect a growing interest in balancing modern science with ancestral knowledge. The subtlety of selenium's role in culture mirrors its often understated, yet essential, function in human health.

Perhaps one of the more intriguing aspects of gold and selenium is how they've transcended their original cultural boundaries to influence contemporary alternative medicine practices worldwide. Today, proponents of alternative medicine advocate for the therapeutic potential of these elements, drawing connections between ancient beliefs and modern health practices. The idea of gold as a miraculous healer has seen a resurgence, with some contemporary wellness circles extolling its virtues in promoting both physical and mental well-being.

The use of gold and selenium in alternative medicine varies significantly across the globe, largely shaped by each culture's heritage and worldview. In parts of Asia and Africa, gold is still believed to possess a healing energy, akin to chi or prana, underpinning its use in holistic health practices. These views are often tied to a broader narrative that sees health as an integration of body, mind, and spirit—a perspective that can't easily be compartmentalized into Western medical paradigms.

Turning to selenium, cultural applications are emerging more visibly in regions where research is uncovering its health benefits. In countries like Brazil and Japan, known for their comprehensive approaches to health and wellness, selenium is increasingly being incorporated into dietary supplements and functional foods. This embrace of selenium highlights a cultural shift towards valuing preventive health measures, offering a contrast to other regions where reactive treatment still predominates.

The global landscape of gold and selenium usage also reveals a tapestry of beliefs around purity and poison. While gold is almost universally regarded as a symbol of purity and incorruptibility, its alchemical associations have steered some cultures towards caution, wary of the fine line between cure and toxicity. Similarly, while selenium's antioxidant properties are celebrated, its potential toxicity when mishandled is a sobering reminder of nature's duality. Thus, understanding cultural practices involves not only looking at how these elements are utilized but also how their risks are perceived and managed.

As we delve deeper into these cultural perspectives, it becomes clear that both gold and selenium occupy an intersection of faith, science, and tradition. Their roles in healing are debated and refined over time, reflecting changes in cultural attitudes and scientific understandings. For the health-conscious individual or medical professional exploring these elements, recognizing cultural contexts is essential. It enriches the dialogue between conventional and alternative medicine, fostering a more holistic appreciation of wellness.

In many ways, the cultural practices surrounding gold and selenium illustrate a broader human inclination for balance and harmony. Whether in traditional Chinese medicine or Ayurvedic traditions, the quest is not merely for cure but for a deeper state of equilibrium with nature. This cultural wisdom offers a poignant reminder that in the pursuit of health, understanding the past is as crucial as embracing the future.

In summation, the cultural views and practices around gold and selenium provide a multifaceted lens through which to view these elements beyond their scientific properties. They invite a consideration of how traditions shape our understanding and usage of natural resources, encouraging a dialogue between history, culture, and medicine. For those who seek to investigate and inform, these cultural perspectives offer a treasure trove of insights, underscoring the profound interconnectedness of our global community.

International Case Studies

The use of gold and selenium in medicine is not confined within borders; it's a global exploration, rich with varied case studies that highlight differing approaches and outcomes. Across the world, researchers and practitioners have applied these elements in treating diseases and enhancing well-being, with each region reflecting its unique cultural and scientific backdrop. This section delves into international case studies that illuminate the fascinating tapestry of global health perspectives on gold and selenium.

In India, for example, the integration of gold in traditional Ayurvedic practices has been long-standing. Known locally as "Swarn Bhasma," gold ash has been used in rejuvenation therapies aimed at boosting immunity and improving mental capabilities. Recent studies conducted in collaboration with Western medical facilities aim to scientifically validate these traditional uses. One fascinating study observed patients with rheumatoid arthritis receiving gold therapy in varying dosages, with many participants reporting significant improvement in joint pain and swelling.

Meanwhile, in Brazil, selenium's role in health has been predominantly researched concerning its impact on thyroid function. As a country with regions rich in selenium due to natural soil content, Brazil has been pivotal in studying how selenium supplementation impacts thyroid health. A study focusing on Brazilian regions with varying selenium concentrations in the soil offered insights into the prevention of thyroid diseases, specifically Hashimoto's thyroiditis. The findings suggested that residents in selenium-rich areas had lower incidences of thyroid dysfunction, sparking interest in using selenium as a preventive measure globally.

In Japan, the practice of integrating gold in skincare and anti-aging products has become a substantial industry. This fascination with gold goes beyond luxury and into the realm of cellular regeneration. Researchers in Tokyo are conducting controlled clinical trials to ascertain the potential for gold nanoparticles to accelerate skin healing processes. These studies might lead to breakthroughs in cosmetic and medical dermatology treatments worldwide.

Across Europe, selenium's potential in cancer prevention is a hot topic. The Swedish Selenium Prevention Study, which involved over a thousand participants, found varying degrees of success in reducing prostate cancer risks when selenium supplements were introduced. The study's rigorous methodology and promising results have set a precedent for European health policies considering selenium as an essential dietary supplement for cancer prevention.

In Africa, where infectious diseases pose a significant health challenge, research on the combined effects of gold and selenium has been emerging. In Ghana, a pilot program exploring these elements' nutritional supplementation is being conducted among populations affected by malaria. Preliminary results indicate potential health benefits, including reduced oxidative stress and improved immune responses, though more expansive research is necessary to confirm these findings.

Chinese medicine has a long history of using minerals in treatment formulas. Here, gold is often integrated with other herbs to enhance its therapeutic properties in treating conditions like insomnia and anxiety. Modern Chinese hospitals are now conducting integrated studies using traditional methods supplemented with insights from Western science. These hybrid studies aim to offer evidence-based recommendations that could harmonize traditional practices with modern medical protocols.

Australia offers another unique viewpoint; it's at the forefront of researching selenium's role in skin cancer prevention, reflecting the country's high incidence of skin cancer. The University of Sydney's longitudinal study tracks the effects of daily selenium supplementation on skin cancer rates. This initiative is part of a larger effort to establish preventative strategies in regions with high sun exposure.

Transitioning to the Middle East, Israel's exploration of gold in medicine has led to innovative research, particularly in the context of targeted cancer therapies. The Hebrew University in Jerusalem is currently investigating the use of gold nanoparticles as a delivery system for chemotherapy drugs. Early results are promising, indicating improved targeting and reduced side effects compared to traditional chemotherapy methods.

Lastly, Russia has been revisiting selenium's role following their study on residents around the Ural Mountains, where selenium deficiencies have been linked to increased risks of cardiovascular diseases. The Russian Academy of Sciences is now spearheading a project that incorporates selenium supplementation in dietary guidelines in these areas. The goal is to establish if regular selenium intake could significantly reduce the incidence of such diseases.

These international case studies collectively underscore the myriad ways gold and selenium are employed in medical practices across the globe. They highlight the importance of contextual research, often influenced by regional health challenges, cultural practices, and available natural resources. As these studies continue to develop, they pave the way for a broader understanding and potential integration of these elements into mainstream health paradigms, challenging traditional boundaries and encouraging a more holistic approach to health and wellness. The global perspectives offered here open doors to new possibilities, showcasing the diversity and innovation present in the intersection of culture and science.

Chapter 21: Implementing Holistic Approaches

As the discussion around alternative medicine gains momentum, implementing holistic approaches is fast becoming an essential strategy in comprehensive healthcare. Bridging various treatment modalities isn't just about stacking remedies; it's a meticulous orchestration of therapies that attend to the body, mind, and spirit simultaneously. In the realm of gold and selenium treatments, integrating holistic methods can bolster patient resilience, enhance the efficacy of primary treatments, and mitigate side effects. The synergy of nutrition, emotional support, and traditional medicine crafts a palette of care that is as dynamic as it is personalized. Exploring these complex interactions involves not only scientific rigor but also an embracing of medical intuition, creating a dialogue where empirical evidence and patient narratives coexist. This chapter delves into strategies that weave together diverse healing practices, nudging the boundaries of what is conventionally accepted in medical circles, all while maintaining a keen eye on safety and efficacy.

Comprehensive Care Strategies

In the pursuit of optimal health, there's an emerging recognition of the need for comprehensive care strategies. These approaches aren't just about treating symptoms or diseases superficially; they're about diving deeper, looking at the whole picture of a patient's well-being. This involves integrating different modalities and therapies to support an individual physically, mentally, emotionally, and sometimes even spiritually. The aim is to create a system where conventional and alternative treatments work in unison, offering holistic benefits that singular approaches may miss.

Consider the principle of individualization in care. It's crucial in the landscape of holistic approaches, as each person's health journey is unique. Tailoring treatment plans that consider the individual's life circumstances, medical history, genetic predispositions, and emotional states leads to more effective care. By embracing personalized medicine, medical professionals can create more precise interventions. This strategy often involves a combination of mainstream treatments, dietary modifications, supplementation such as gold and selenium, exercise regimens, and stress management techniques.

Interestingly, the rise of integrative medicine reflects a broader trend toward health paradigms that see the individual as a complete system. When implementing this approach, clinicians and health practitioners are increasingly utilizing practices like acupuncture, chiropractic care, and mindfulness therapies. These are designed to complement conventional medical treatments. Energy healing, although contentious in some circles, is another frontier being explored. Each therapy aims to enhance the body's natural healing processes, potentially reducing the reliance on pharmaceuticals and invasive procedures.

Interdisciplinary Collaboration: In pursuing comprehensive care strategies, collaboration is key. An interdisciplinary approach leverages the strengths and expertise of various health disciplines, ensuring that patients receive a balanced and nuanced treatment plan. Imagine a team where oncologists, nutritionists, psychologists, and alternative medicine practitioners all work together, exploring the best pathways for healing. This collaboration requires open communication, respect for each discipline's contributions, and a robust framework for managing and updating treatment plans as patient needs evolve.

Moreover, such strategies need to be supported by robust scientific data. Research underpins any successful integration of holistic practices. Therefore, ongoing studies and clinical trials are essential to assess the efficacy and safety of combining treatments, such as the synergistic effects of gold and selenium mentioned earlier in this work. Peer-reviewed publications and anecdotal evidence from patient experiences both play critical roles in shaping these holistic strategies, offering insight and validation.

Maintaining a patient-centered approach is at the heart of comprehensive care strategies. Active patient engagement and education empower individuals to take charge of their health journey. This process starts by informing them about the available treatment options, potential benefits, and risks, as well as facilitating informed decision-making. Involving patients in planning and goal-setting fosters a partnership rather than a passive doctor-patient relationship. This approach has been shown to improve adherence to treatment plans and overall satisfaction with care.

Nutrition often serves as a cornerstone in comprehensive care strategies. It's not merely a matter of fad diets or supplement stacks. Instead, it's about understanding how food and nutrition interact with one's biochemistry, thereby influencing health outcomes. Targeted nutrition involves the strategic inclusion of foods and supplements like those containing selenium and organic compounds. These can expedite the healing process or play preventative roles in conditions such as cancer and other chronic illnesses.

The mental and emotional dimensions of healing cannot be underestimated. Strategies that incorporate cognitive-behavioral therapies, meditation, and even artistic therapies can enhance psychological resilience and reduce stress. The mind-body connection is an area that continues to gain credibility in medical circles, supported by research into how psychological states can impact physical health and recovery outcomes.

Barrier-breaking technology also provides new avenues to support comprehensive care strategies. These include mobile health apps, telemedicine platforms, and wearable health monitors. They play a vital role in patient monitoring, offering real-time data that can inform treatment adjustments promptly. Access to such technology allows for enhanced engagement and compliance, giving patients the tools they need to actively manage their health outside of traditional medical settings.

Ultimately, implementing holistic approaches calls for an intricate balancing act. It's about weighing the benefits of traditinal and alternative practices, recognizing the unique journey of each patient, and above all, maintaining the integrity of care through evidence-based practices. As health perspectives continue to expand and embrace holistic paradigms, comprehensive care strategies hold the promise of a more responsive and patient-aligned future in medicine. Such strategies not only treat illness but cultivate a state of wellness that can sustain individuals over the long term.

Integrating Multiple Treatments

In the ever-evolving world of medicine, the conversation is shifting from single-solution therapies to a more integrated approach to patient care. Holistic methodologies advocate for treating the patient as a whole, rather than compartmentalizing care into distinct and separate actions. This strategy stems from the realization that illnesses seldom impact just one aspect of a person's health. Therefore, the integration of multiple treatments becomes not only beneficial but imperative.

At its core, integrating different therapeutic strategies means bringing together the best of all worlds—conventional medicine and alternative practices—creating a cohesive treatment strategy tailored to each individual's needs. Historically, Western medicine has prioritized a symptom-centric approach, often focusing on treating the most immediate and visible aspects of illness. Alternative medicines, meanwhile, lend themselves to a more preventative and long-term form of care.

The benefits of a multimodal approach are numerous. By using a variety of treatments, patients receive a well-rounded treatment plan that addresses physical, mental, and emotional health aspects. This is particularly effective for chronic conditions where multiple system involvements need to be considered. For example, cancer treatment often necessitates chemotherapy, radiation, and surgery—methods rooted in traditional Western medicine. However, integrating methods like acupuncture, nutrition-based therapy, and meditation can support the physical and emotional endurance required in these treatments.

Nonetheless, developing a comprehensive treatment plan requires careful consideration and strategic planning. Diverse practices need to be harmonized to ensure they work synergistically rather than contradict each other. Coordination among healthcare providers is essential, which can be achieved through meticulous communication and documentation. Modern electronic health records provide a platform for practitioners from varying disciplines to access shared information, ensuring seamless integration.

Such integrative strategies aren't without challenges. Aligning traditional and alternative treatments can face skepticism from practitioners entrenched in their respective fields. Yet, bridging the gap between these worlds has the potential to enhance patient outcomes significantly. Some medical professionals may worry about the efficacy of alternative methods or potential interactions with standard treatments. Counterbalancing these concerns involves rigorous and continued scientific research. Studies investigating the synergy between different treatments, such as the use of monoatomic gold and selenium, are vital in alleviating these apprehensions.

It's also crucial to acknowledge the patient's role in integrating multiple treatments. Empowering patients with information allows them to make informed decisions about their care. This shared decision-making process requires transparency, with practitioners communicating both the benefits and risks associated with each treatment option. Patients who fully understand and participate in their treatment plan adhere better and are more likely to see positive outcomes.

Healthcare systems that support integrated treatment models should prioritize training for medical practitioners in alternative interventions, ensuring they are well-versed in both conventional and non-conventional therapies. This includes fostering a collaborative spirit within healthcare teams and encouraging openness to diverse practices. Furthermore, research should continue to explore successful case studies wherein integrated treatments have achieved remarkable results.

Ultimately, the integration of multiple treatments can transform the healthcare landscape. In a world where patients demand more personalized care options tailored to their unique conditions, this holistic approach holds promise. Refusing to treat symptoms in isolation and instead focusing on the patient's overall wellbeing is a significant step forward in modern medicine.

Chapter 22: Myths and Misconceptions

When it comes to alternative medicine, particularly the use of substances like gold and selenium, myths and misconceptions thrive. Common yet consequential misbeliefs can lead to both undue skepticism and misplaced confidence. Let's unravel these myths by highlighting scientific clarifications. For instance, while monoatomic gold is often touted as a miraculous cure-all, scientific support for such claims is scant. Misunderstandings about selenium's role in health also abound. It's crucial for health-conscious individuals and medical professionals to discern fact from fiction, approaching these treatments with an investigative mindset. Persuasive yet grounded narratives can lead to informed decisions. Myth-busting isn't just about setting records straight; it's about encouraging skeptical inquiry and fostering a more nuanced understanding of alternative treatments.

Debunking Common Myths

In the vast landscape of health and wellness, myths take root easily, often masquerading as truths through repetition and anecdote. While some of these myths offer comforting narratives, they can obscure reality and mislead those seeking genuine solutions. When it comes to alternative treatments involving monoatomic gold and selenium, the myths run deep. They propagate misconceptions that can influence health decisions, making it crucial to sift through the noise for clarity and accuracy.

One prevalent myth is that monoatomic gold has mystical properties that can cure diseases instantly. While this makes an enticing story, it's far from substantiated by current scientific evidence. The notion often stems from ancient beliefs associated with gold's perceived sacredness and its use by alchemists. Today, without rigorous studies to validate such claims, relying on monoatomic gold as a miracle cure is more wishful thinking than fact. It is important to approach health interventions with a critical eye, seeking substantiation rather than succumbing to the allure of ancient allurements.

Another common misconception is that all natural treatments, because they are 'natural', are inherently safe. While selenium is an essential nutrient, significant in small doses for maintaining certain bodily functions, excessive intake can lead to toxicity. This misunderstood threshold between benefit and harm is often glossed over in discussions promoting alternative treatments. The danger lies in self-prescribing what is commonly perceived as harmless due to its natural origin. Therefore, proper dosage and professional guidance should not be disregarded.

The idea that combining gold and selenium can catapult one to optimal health status is another myth needing attention. While studies delve into the biochemical interactions between these elements, the synergy is not a blanket solution for health issues. Complex conditions like cancer or chronic illnesses require multifaceted treatment approaches rather than singular, unproven remedies. It's essential to understand that biochemical investigations, while promising, do not always translate to unequivocal clinical success.

Some advocates claim that monoatomic gold can improve spiritual or cognitive functions. This claim often leans heavily on individual testimonies rather than scientific rigor. The placebo effect can sometimes be misconstrued as real benefit, occasionally leading individuals to believe in enhancements that are more psychological than physiological. This is where an understanding of scientific methodology, the distinction between anecdote and evidence, becomes paramount.

The advent of misinformation via digital platforms further perpetuates these myths. Clickbait headlines and viral social media posts can spread false narratives rapidly, leading people to accept unsupported claims as truths. In this information age, distinguishing credible information from noise demands a skeptical mindset and a thorough evaluation of sources. Critical thinking and fact-checking must be at the forefront of any health-related inquiry.

A recurring myth is that alternative therapies, such as those involving gold and selenium, are actively suppressed by mainstream medicine due to pharmaceutical interests. This oversimplifies the complex interplay between alternative and conventional medicine. While it is true that the pharmaceutical industry holds significant power, it is incorrect to assume neglect of alternative methods solely as a barrier to profit. Every treatment, alternative or traditional, should aim to meet rigorous standards for safety and efficacy.

It is equally misguided to believe that all negative reports about these alternative treatments are part of an elaborate conspiracy to discredit them. On the contrary, scientific scrutiny is a necessary mechanism to ensure patient safety and effective treatment options. Peer-reviewed studies, though not infallible, provide a more objective assessment when compared to individual experiences or biased narratives.

Lastly, there's a myth advocating that relying solely on alternative treatments, dismissing modern medicine altogether, is a viable health strategy. This dichotomy between natural and pharmaceutical remedies promotes an either/or mindset that isn't where healing should reside. Integrative approaches, blending the strengths of both spheres, offer a more balanced and potentially effective pathway to health. It is about finding harmony rather than conflict between traditional and alternative paradigms.

In conclusion, debunking these myths requires a rigorous application of skepticism and a willingness to engage with evidence over hearsay. In the quest for optimal health, challenges arise when misinformation skews reality. Understanding these myths, dissecting their origins and implications, provides clarity. This knowledge empowers individuals to make informed choices, marrying curiosity with caution, and virtue with validation. It's a journey towards truth, grounded in evidence, stripped of illusion, and focused on the genuine pursuit of wellness.

Scientific Clarifications

The world of alternative medicine often swims in a sea of myths and misconceptions, particularly when it comes to the use of substances like gold and selenium. Sometimes it feels like these discussions are floating between the realms of plausible science and fantastical alchemy. When myths propagate, they often muddy the waters of scientific understanding, requiring rigorous clarification. We must separate the wheat from the chaff and focus on evidence-based assessments.

One of the first clarifications concerns monoatomic gold, which is often surrounded by miraculous claims. Some suggest that it can promote spiritual enlightenment or even extend lifespan. However, from a scientific standpoint, there is no peer-reviewed evidence substantiating these extravagant claims. Monoatomic elements, especially in the context of health benefits, appear to dwell more in the realm of speculation than in validated science.

An important question is often posed: What does the science say about the application of gold and selenium in conventional medicine? The literature as it stands is clear: Both substances hold potential, yet their application is far from universally understood. Gold compounds, for example, have been used in the treatment of rheumatoid arthritis, underlining the specific conditions where they have validated therapeutic value. They work by moderating immune responses, but their function is distinct and highly targeted, a far cry from the mythical cure-all some propose.

Selenium, on the other hand, finds itself in a slightly different position. It is an essential micronutrient, critical for several physiological processes such as thyroid hormone metabolism and antioxidant defense systems. While its role in preventing diseases such as cancer has been studied, the results are often mixed. Selenium deficiency does correlate with certain health problems, but excessive supplementation can be toxic, illustrating the importance of balance and precision in its use.

We must also dive into the biochemical interactions between gold and selenium, as there's a burgeoning interest in their synergistic effects. Studies suggest that when used together, they may enhance each other's efficacy in specific medical contexts, such as cancer treatment. Nevertheless, these studies are still in exploratory stages, and it would be premature to make significant conclusions without more robust clinical trials that thoroughly verify safety and effectiveness.

Further scientific clarification arises when discussing alchemy's modern resurgence. While alchemy provides a fascinating historical context, today's scientific methodologies demand rigorous testing and evidence that transcends mystical associations. Modern biochemistry and molecular biology have the tools to demystify such practices, rigorously investigating any claim before it's integrated into mainstream medicine. Thus, sites where modern science meets ancient practice often require not just more data but more significant oversight.

Scientific research methodologies play a crucial role in busting myths. The integrity of a scientific study lies in its methodology – randomization, blinding, peer review process, and sample size, to name a few essentials. Distilling reliable conclusions from unfounded claims requires a great deal of skepticism and a commitment to evidence. Clinical trials, when conducted without bias and with proper controls, can shed light on whether a treatment's perceived benefits are due to the treatment itself or merely a placebo effect.

Another layer of clarification involves the skepticism and criticisms often directed at alternative treatments. While skepticism can lead to valuable insights, unyielding criticism may sometimes leave valid benefits unexplored. Here lies the importance of an open yet critically evaluative approach to new findings in the use of gold and selenium. For alternative treatments to gain wider acceptance, they must face the same scientific scrutiny as any conventional treatment.

It's essential to address the risks and possible side effects commonly associated with alternative substances. Many people believe consuming these elements in any quantity offers health benefits. This belief is misleading. It's crucial to emphasize the importance of dosage and the conditions under which these substances can be safely administered. Overconsumption or contamination can seriously harm one's health.

The myths surrounding these substances often spread quickly without scientific backing, largely due to persuasive anecdotes and testimonials. While personal stories can be compelling and emotionally resonant, they seldom hold the weight of scientific validation. The power of anecdotal evidence should not be downplayed, but it needs to be carefully balanced with scientific research.

As we continue to explore the intersection of gold and selenium's potential health benefits, we return to the core scientific principles that guide responsible investigation. Each claim must undergo rigorous testing before being accepted into the landscape of validated medical treatments. There's a wealth of potential in these elements, but realizing that potential responsibly is a journey fueled by strict adherence to scientific integrity.

Ultimately, by continually critiquing methods, questioning results, and refining understandings, science offers the clearest pathway through the fog of misinformation. Through this lens, myths and misconceptions can be effectively dispelled, paving the way for genuine advancements in both alternative and conventional medicine. This reflective examination of evidence ensures that true scientific marvels, rather than fanciful mythologies, define our understanding of monoatomic gold and selenium.

Chapter 23: The Role of Technology in Research

Technology is increasingly shaping the landscape of medical research, especially in exploring alternative medicine solutions like gold and selenium. Advanced tools such as AI algorithms and machine learning transform data analysis, allowing researchers to uncover patterns and correlations that were previously obscured by complex variables. These innovations don't just push the boundaries of what's possible; they also democratize research, making it accessible to a wider range of medical professionals and institutions. For health-conscious individuals and medical experts alike, technology offers a double-edged sword of piquing curiosity and demanding skepticism. As wearable devices track health markers in real-time, researchers can gain insights into the long-term effects of alternative treatments that were once speculative. However, the rapid pace of technological advancement also poses challenges, underscoring the need for rigorous peer review and ethical considerations to ensure that these powerful tools are used wisely. Thus, technology is not merely an enabler of research; it is a catalyst that provokes critical thought and innovation in understanding and harnessing alternative health solutions.

Advanced Tools and Techniques

In the expanding field of research, especially concerning alternative medicine, technology has become an indispensable ally. As we delve deeper into the intricacies of gold and selenium's roles in health and treatment, it's crucial to recognize the technological advancements paving this path. These advanced tools are not merely apparatus but act as catalysts, expediting the exploration of complex biochemical processes and enabling scientists to unravel the mysteries that have baffled humanity for centuries.

The advent of high-throughput screening has revolutionized the field. This method allows researchers to simultaneously test thousands of samples against potential therapeutic agents, such as gold and selenium. By doing so, it accelerates the discovery process, identifying viable leads faster than traditional methods. What used to take years or even decades to uncover can now be achieved in months. High-throughput screening doesn't just speed up the process; it enhances accuracy, providing reliable data that researchers can build upon.

Moreover, computational modeling and simulations have become pivotal. These techniques enable researchers to create complex models of molecular interactions on digital platforms. With computational power, scientists can simulate how selenium and gold might interact at a cellular level under various biological conditions. This capability not only saves time and resources but also allows researchers to toggle variables and observe potential outcomes without physical experimentation. It's like running countless 'what-if' scenarios in a virtual lab setting, honing in on the most promising paths for further investigation.

In conjunction with these methods, bioinformatics has emerged as a critical component of modern research. Leveraging vast databases, bioinformatics facilitates the analysis and interpretation of complex biological data. When it comes to gold and selenium, this can mean unraveling genetic expressions affected by these elements and understanding their potential impacts on diseases like cancer. By sifting through data, researchers can identify patterns and correlations that might not be immediately evident, opening up new avenues for exploration.

Emerging technologies such as CRISPR-Cas9, the revolutionary gene-editing tool, have also been instrumental. While primarily known for its applications in genetics, CRISPR's precision in modifying genetic codes has vast implications in understanding the therapeutic potential of gold and selenium. Researchers can edit genes within cells to observe how changes affect reactions to these elements, deepening the understanding of their roles and potentially guiding personalized medicine strategies.

The power of artificial intelligence (AI) and machine learning cannot be overstated. These technologies are transforming how we conduct research by identifying patterns and predicting outcomes with remarkable speed and accuracy. AI can analyze large datasets to determine outcomes of various treatments involving gold and selenium, providing insights that would be daunting, if not impossible, for humans to extract manually. Machine learning algorithms continuously improve, learning from new data to refine predictions and offer more targeted solutions in the pursuit of effective treatments.

Beyond the laboratory, technology also plays a pivotal role in disseminating findings and fostering collaboration among researchers worldwide. Cloud-based platforms and data-sharing networks have created a global symposium of sorts, where scientists can share their findings, access peer studies, and collaborate in real-time. This global connectivity ensures that discoveries and advancements in the use of gold and selenium are swiftly communicated, avoiding duplication of efforts and fostering a more integrated approach to research challenges.

Laboratory technology, including advanced spectrometry and electron microscopy, permits researchers to view the minutest details of biological interactions. For instance, gold nanoparticles' interaction at the cellular level can be visualized in great detail, offering insights into their mechanisms of action. These tools allow a glimpse into the cellular 'dance,' showing how gold and selenium integrate within biological systems, providing a clearer picture of their therapeutic potential.

Furthermore, wearable technology has extended the frontier of research from laboratories to everyday life. Devices that track vital statistics can provide real-time data on how individuals respond to treatments involving gold and selenium. Continuous monitoring opens new doors in understanding the personalized effects of these elements, potentially leading to more tailored and effective treatment protocols.

While the integration of these advanced tools and techniques in research is palpable, it is imperative to remain vigilant about ethical considerations and potential pitfalls. With great power comes the responsibility to ensure that technology serves the betterment of humanity and not merely the pursuit of scientific curiosity. The tools at our disposal must be wielded with care, a lesson history has taught us repeatedly. As we continue to explore the ramifications of gold and selenium in alternative medicine, these technological advancements provide both the map and the compass.

Looking forward, the synergy between technology and medical research will only deepen. Technology will continue to evolve, and with it, our ability to decipher the complex roles of elements like gold and selenium in promoting health and healing. In uncovering hidden truths, we not only advance our understanding but also pay homage to those who have treaded the path before us, driven by the same quest for knowledge and a better tomorrow.

Innovative Research Methods

As we delve into the intricacies of the role of technology in research, we can't overlook how innovative research methods have reshaped our understanding of various fields, including alternative medicine. The integration of advanced technological tools and novel methodologies has opened new avenues for exploration and discovery. This section seeks to illuminate how these pioneering techniques are being employed to investigate the potential of treatments such as those involving gold and selenium.

One of the most transformative aspects of modern research is the shift towards data-driven methodologies. In the context of health research, especially in alternative treatments, there's a newfound emphasis on harnessing big data analytics. By analyzing massive datasets, researchers can identify patterns and correlations that were previously hidden. This approach not only aids in understanding the efficacy of treatments but also plays a crucial role in uncovering potential risks associated with them.

Machine learning algorithms, a subset of artificial intelligence, are increasingly being utilized to predict outcomes and personalize treatment approaches. These algorithms can process vast amounts of information, learning from patient histories, genetic data, and treatment responses to suggest optimal treatment plans tailored to individual needs. Imagine a world where technology predicts which patients might benefit the most from gold or selenium supplements in their treatment regimen, optimizing therapeutic outcomes while minimizing side effects.

Moving beyond the realm of data analysis, innovative research methods also encompass advancements in laboratory techniques. The use of nanoscale technologies, like nanomedicine, is particularly promising. It enables scientists to create nanoparticles of gold that can be used in drug delivery systems—possibly increasing the effectiveness and precision of treatments. This method represents a convergence of traditional healing substances with cutting-edge technology, offering a glimpse into the future of personalized medicine.

In vivo testing, although traditional, has also undergone significant transformations with the advent of new tools. Today, imaging techniques such as advanced MRI and PET scans allow for real-time observation of how substances like selenium interact within the body. These images can be captured with remarkable detail, providing insights into biochemical pathways and the immediate effects of supplements. Such precision helps in refining dosage and understanding the exact mechanisms through which these alternative treatments exert their influence.

Another frontier that's pushing the boundaries of research is the field of bioinformatics. This approach involves the development and application of computational tools to gather, analyze, and interpret complex biological data. For those studying the interplay between gold, selenium, and human biology, bioinformatics offers a way to decode interactions at a molecular level. By mapping out these interactions, researchers can build more robust theories on how to employ these elements for therapeutic benefit.

Furthermore, crowd-sourced platforms and citizen science initiatives exemplify how participation in research has expanded beyond traditional laboratories. These platforms empower individuals, including patients and physicians, to contribute data and insights based on personal experiences. The collective data amassed through such participatory approaches can accelerate research and offer real-world evidence that complements traditional clinical trials.

It's also essential to consider the ethical implications of these innovative methods. While technology offers unprecedented opportunities, it also raises questions about privacy, data security, and consent. Researchers must navigate these waters carefully, ensuring that ethical guidelines are rigorously upheld to maintain public trust and protect participant rights.

Discussing innovative research methods isn't complete without acknowledging the resurgence of multidisciplinary approaches. The convergence of fields like physics, chemistry, biology, and computer science is enabling breakthroughs that were once considered the stuff of science fiction. This collaborative spirit not only accelerates the pace of discovery but also ensures that the findings are robust and applicable across various contexts and cultures.

The adoption of virtual reality (VR) and augmented reality (AR) in research is another testament to innovation. These technologies allow researchers to simulate clinical environments and visualize complex processes in three dimensions. Such simulations can be particularly helpful in educational settings, training medical professionals in alternative treatment protocols that incorporate gold and selenium. Their immersive nature ensures that abstract concepts are made tangible, facilitating better understanding and application.

Lastly, it's important to keep in mind that with rapid technological progress, there is an ongoing need for agile methodologies in research. These methods, which emphasize iterative testing and flexibility, align perfectly with the evolving nature of medical research. In particular, adaptive trial designs allow for modifications to be made as new information becomes available, thereby ensuring that research remains relevant and effective.

In conclusion, innovative research methods powered by technological advancements are redefining the landscape of medical research, especially in the realm of alternative treatments. By leveraging big data, machine learning, bioinformatics, and other technologies, researchers are equipped with powerful tools to investigate and harness the potential of treatments involving gold and selenium. This transformative period in research not only promises enhanced therapeutic outcomes but also challenges us to rethink how we approach scientific inquiries in an interconnected world.

Chapter 24: Health Policy and Community Impacts

The intersection of health policy and alternative medicine is a dynamic space, reshaping communities and sparking profound debate. As alternative treatments like monoatomic gold and selenium gain traction, there is a tangible shift in how communities engage with health resources. Policies often lag behind scientific discoveries, leaving a gap that local advocates strive to fill through grassroots movements. In areas where conventional health services falter, community-driven initiatives utilizing alternative treatments have gained a foothold, transforming lives by fostering inclusive healthcare environments. The success stories that emerge from these communities offer a compelling narrative—one where empowered citizens advocate for policy changes that reflect their diverse health needs. This paradigmal shift challenges policymakers to reconcile evidence-based practices with emerging therapeutic insights, signaling the dawn of a more personalized health landscape where policy and practice are inexorably linked.

Influencing Health Policies

Influencing health policies requires not only scientific evidence but also a concerted effort to align with social values and community needs. In recent years, the intersection of alternative medicine and conventional practices has sparked significant debates across the healthcare landscape. This dialogue has only intensified with the increasing interest in substances like monoatomic gold and selenium. Their potential health benefits, albeit controversial, require a thorough examination of how policies can adapt to incorporate such advancements while ensuring safety and efficacy.

Health policies have a profound impact on the accessibility and integration of alternative treatments within mainstream medical practices. The challenge lies in bridging the gap between empirical research and public acceptance, all while adhering to regulatory frameworks. Controversial treatments often face an uphill battle in gaining broad acceptance, partly due to the skepticism inherent in the scientific community and partly due to legislative hurdles. There is a pressing need for advocates of alternative medicine to engage with policymakers in creating a more inclusive approach to healthcare options.

The process of influencing health policies begins with robust scientific research. Studies that demonstrate the efficacy and safety of treatments are crucial. However, even when such evidence exists, translating it into policy requires a strategic approach. Research findings must be communicated effectively to policymakers, who may not have the expertise to interpret scientific data. Clear, concise communication that highlights the potential benefits, risks, and implications of alternative treatments can pave the way for policy consideration and eventual adoption.

Moreover, stakeholder engagement is vital. Health policy is often shaped by various interest groups, including healthcare providers, pharmaceutical companies, patient advocacy groups, and government agencies. Each of these entities has distinct priorities and concerns. Meaningful dialogue among stakeholders can foster a collaborative environment where diverse perspectives are respected and integrated into policy formulation. By facilitating conversations that emphasize common goals—such as improved patient outcomes and access to diverse treatment options—advocates can influence policy decisions more effectively.

A notable example is the growing recognition of integrative medicine, which combines conventional and alternative approaches to healthcare. Policies supporting integrative practices have emerged in response to increased demand from patients seeking comprehensive care strategies. Such policies underscore the importance of holistic approaches that consider physical, emotional, and social well-being. Integrative medicine represents a model for how alternative treatments can be incorporated into health policies, leading to more personalized and patient-centered care.

Economic factors also play a significant role in shaping health policies. The cost-effectiveness of alternative treatments, such as employing natural supplements instead of expensive pharmaceuticals, can be an appealing argument for policymakers. Financial constraints often drive the need for innovative and sustainable healthcare solutions. Demonstrating that alternative treatments offer financial benefits without compromising quality or safety can bolster efforts to influence policies favorably.

Yet, the transition from research to policy is not without challenges. One major hurdle is the standardization of alternative treatments. For substances like monoatomic gold and selenium, establishing standardized dosages and protocols is essential for ensuring consistent and reliable outcomes. Lack of standardization can lead to variable results and diminished credibility, which can stall policy developments. Researchers and practitioners must work towards consensus on dosage guidelines to gain the trust of both the public and policymakers.

Additionally, education and awareness play crucial roles in influencing health policies. An informed public is more likely to advocate for policies that align with their health beliefs and experiences. Education campaigns that present alternative treatments in an evidence-based and balanced manner can promote understanding and acceptance. Likewise, educating medical professionals about the potential benefits and limitations of alternative treatments can facilitate an informed discourse on policy development and integration into clinical practice.

The role of advocacy groups cannot be underestimated in the policy-making process. These groups often serve as a bridge between the public and policymakers, lobbying for changes that reflect emerging health trends and patient needs. Effective advocacy involves not only presenting scientific data but also sharing compelling narratives that resonate with policymakers on a personal level. Testimonials from individuals who have benefitted from alternative treatments often underscore the human impact of policy decisions and can be powerful catalysts for change.

Looking forward, the future of health policy in relation to alternative treatments hinges on adaptability and openness to innovation. Policymakers must be willing to consider new evidence and adjust policies accordingly. This requires an environment of trust and cooperation, where scientific evidence is not only available but also actively sought and integrated into decision-making processes.

Ultimately, influencing health policies is a dynamic and multifaceted endeavor. It requires a balance between scientific rigor and social advocacy, between addressing current healthcare challenges and anticipating future needs. By fostering a collaborative spirit among researchers, clinicians, policymakers, and the community, we can pave the way for a more inclusive, effective, and responsive healthcare system. This can ensure that both conventional and alternative treatments are explored to their fullest potential, offering patients the best possible outcomes.

Community Success Stories

As healthcare paradigms shift towards integrating traditional and alternative practices, communities around the world are witnessing remarkable success stories. These narratives aren't just about individuals finding solace in alternative treatments; they are about communities redefining health boundaries and perceptions collectively. The grassroots impact of such stories is significant, as they breathe life into dry statistics and clinical trials, translating complex data into everyday language and experiences.

Take, for instance, a small town in Arizona where residents have integrated selenium-rich foods and monoatomic gold supplementation into their community health programs. This grassroots initiative was sparked by a group of local healthcare providers who were keen on pursuing holistic approaches. They embarked on this journey not just through introducing these elements but by advocating for a complete lifestyle revamp. Community events focused on education, cooking demonstrations, and wellness clinics not only informed the public but actively engaged them in learning about the benefits and potential of alternative treatments. The result? A marked improvement in community health metrics, notably in areas like immune function and energy levels.

Elsewhere, in the coastal villages of Maine, fishermen who turned to alternative treatments after suffering from occupational health issues report an unexpected revitalization. With arthritis and joint problems being prevalent due to their demanding careers, they were introduced to a novel combination of diet changes involving selenium and therapies that included gold-based ointments. Initially met with skepticism, word of mouth soon turned this approach into a village-wide initiative, significantly reducing absenteeism and enhancing quality of life scores among the residents.

A key aspect of these success stories is the impact of community involvement and peer support. In a tight-knit community, once a few individuals share positive experiences, it propels others to follow suit. This collective momentum often leads to more structured community health initiatives and pushes local policymakers to consider alternative treatments more seriously. Furthermore, these stories highlight the importance of not just individual health outcomes but collective community well-being. When a community adopts a health initiative en masse, it can create a support system that aids in adherence and provides encouragement through shared experiences.

In contrast, urban areas offer a different kind of success story narrative, often revolving around diversity and innovation. In San Francisco, a city brimming with heterogeneity, the cultural adaptability towards alternative treatments has been significantly shaped by its diverse population. Various communities have tailored alternative treatment programs that align with their cultural values and medical beliefs, blending elements like monoatomic gold into culturally sensitive healthcare practices. This adaptive innovation has fostered a spirit of embracing the future of medicine while respecting age-old traditions. Moreover, it has opened avenues for cross-cultural exchanges of medical practices, creating a melting pot of ideas and solutions.

An equally intriguing example is seen in Florida, where a retirement community has taken the mantle to explore alternative treatments holistically. Recognizing the limitations of conventional approaches to age-related ailments, they initiated a participatory program focused on treating ailments such as osteoporosis and heart disease with non-traditional therapies involving gold and selenium. The program's design emphasized personalized treatments, incorporating individual dietary preferences and health conditions. The anecdotal evidence of improved vitality and reduced dependency on pharmaceuticals from this community has piqued the interest of both local health authorities and academic researchers, prompting further investigations.

What these stories underscore is not just the potential efficacy of treatments like selenium and monoatomic gold but also the power of collective human experience in healthcare. They shine a light on how public perception can shift when communities actively engage in understanding and experimenting with health interventions. These narratives build a bridge between anecdotal evidence and clinical research, giving researchers a reason to delve deeper into mechanisms that underpin these observed benefits.

While each community's journey with these alternative practices is distinct, their stories share a common thread: the triumph over skepticism and fear of the unfamiliar. Many have defied traditional beliefs, opening doors to alternative treatments, which has often led to improved community health. Success stories become a beacon, a source of inspiration, and a living testament to what is possible when communities dare to step into the unknown and trust in holistic approaches.

Such transformative stories also highlight the critical role of education and awareness in catalyzing change. It isn't merely about access to alternative treatments but involves a deep understanding of their implications, benefits, and limitations. Community workshops, seminars, and health fairs play a significant role in demystifying alternative treatments, removing the stigma and apprehension surrounding them. With increased education, community members become informed advocates, fostering an environment where informed decisions lead to healthcare empowerment.

Beyond any single community, these success stories are reshaping the landscape of health policy discussions. As anecdotal evidence gains traction, there is a growing demand for policies that support further research and integration of alternative treatments into mainstream healthcare. This shift in policy is as much about addressing public demand as it is about recognizing the diverse paths to health and healing. When policymakers witness undeniable benefits arising from community initiatives, they are often compelled to reconsider and adapt healthcare frameworks to be more inclusive of unconventional methods.

In summary, community success stories are more than mere anecdotes; they are a powerful testament to what is achievable when communities come together to explore alternative health solutions. They provide a human face to the often impersonal world of healthcare research and policy, reinforcing the notion that health is not just about the absence of disease but the presence of a thriving, engaged, and informed community. As health-conscious individuals, medical professionals, and those intrigued by alternative medicine solutions continue to listen and learn from these stories, the hope is that they serve as catalysts for broader acceptance and integration of alternative treatments in healthcare.

Chapter 25: Compiling the Evidence

As we reach the crux of our investigation into alternative medicine solutions, the task of compiling the evidence about monoatomic gold and selenium takes center stage. It's a meticulous process, blending meticulous scientific research with narratives from those who've treaded this unconventional path. Building a comprehensive case requires navigating through a mosaic of clinical data, historical accounts, and personal testimonies—each piece shedding light on these elements' potential impacts on health. We aim to bridge the often-gaping chasm between anecdotal claims and empirical validation. This synthesis isn't merely about collecting facts; it's about painting a broader picture—one that may influence future health approaches. As the curtain draws on our exploration, the critical question remains: can we substantiate these alternative claims with enough rigor to push the boundaries of conventional medicine? The crossroads we're at challenges us to consider both what is possible and what is provable. Ultimately, this chapter seeks not only to inform but to ignite dialogue within both the scientific community and among health-conscious individuals about the viability of these intriguing remedies.

Synthesizing Research and Anecdotes

As we delve into the synthesis of research and anecdotes, one must appreciate the deft balancing act between empirical evidence and personal narratives. Capturing the essence of comprehensive understanding is like piecing together a complex puzzle; each study, each patient story is a fragment contributing to a broader picture. It's essential to remember that while research often seeks to generalize findings, anecdotes bring the focus back to individual experiences, enriching the dataset with nuances and variability.

The interplay between quantitative data and qualitative stories is particularly fascinating when evaluating alternative treatments, such as those involving monoatomic gold and selenium. Consider the rigorous methodology of clinical trials—they aim to draw conclusions through structured, reproducible procedures that eliminate bias and enhance reliability. Yet, these structured frameworks sometimes miss the subtle yet significant human experiences documented in patient anecdotes. Here lies the equilibrium that synthesis seeks to achieve, providing a foundation to inform, investigate, and provoke thoughtful discussion.

Scientific literature often provides a robust repository of data, highlighting elements like statistical significance and reproducibility. By comparing results across studies, researchers can establish patterns that are crucial for reliable conclusions. However, when we integrate anecdotal evidence, the result is a tapestry that's richer in texture and depth. It's not just about how many patients responded to a treatment but understanding why some did in unexpected ways, and what that might mean for future research and practice.

The amalgamation of both research and anecdotes becomes particularly important in the realm of alternative medicine, where empirical and personal paths frequently diverge. Evidence-based medicine commands a certain authority; it relies on the aggregation of data across numerous trials and meta-analyses to establish standard clinical practice. But when it comes to uncharted territories where traditional methods meet alternative ones, single officious tones of authority can be more of a barrier than a bridge.

For instance, evaluating the use of monoatomic gold, a less conventional treatment, requires sifting through sparse data and numerous individual stories. Clinical studies might show varying degrees of efficacy, potentially even conflicting results. This can be confusing for health-conscious individuals and medical professionals alike. Anecdotes, meanwhile, offer personal insights— how the treatment affected day-to-day life, unexpected benefits, or, conversely, adverse experiences that might not be fully captured by numbers alone. Together, they provide a more holistic view that resonates with a broader audience.

Anecdotal evidence, while often dismissed as subjective, should not be underestimated. Personal narratives have historically triggered hypotheses that later shaped medical breakthroughs. These stories carry emotional weight and moral urgency, providing context that might not only enhance researchers' hypotheses but could also inspire future studies oriented towards more patient-centered approaches. Such narratives bridge the gap between clinical detachment and humanistic healthcare practices.

Having a comprehensive case where research and anecdotes intertwine involves vivid storytelling backed by data. When we recount a patient's journey using anecdotal evidence, it can be powerful and persuasive. Perhaps a cancer patient combines traditional chemotherapy with selenium supplementation, witnessing incremental yet significant benefits. The individual's story, alongside biochemical studies exploring selenium's role in cancer prevention, offers a relatable backdrop that factual presentations can't achieve on their own.

When discussing how monoatomic gold interacts biochemically within the body, accounts of patients undergoing alternative treatment alongside conventional methods add another layer of understanding and urgency. Such stories might highlight unexpected outcomes: improved energy levels, cognitive clarity, or, crucially, any side effects not evident in clinical metrics. These interactions remind us of medicine's complexity, where human physiology doesn't necessarily adhere to neat, controlled environment assumptions.

Ultimately, the synthesis of research and anecdotes demands an appreciation for both domains. It's an intricate process recognizing that both forms of evidence have their limitations and strengths; neither should be praised nor dismissed outright. The real challenge lies in weaving these strands into a coherent narrative that compels healthcare professionals and patients to view alternative medicine through a lens that values diversity in evidence.

This effort, while labor-intensive, holds significant promise for evolving practice standards. By considering both anecdotal and research-driven insights, medical professionals might develop a more nuanced perspective on alternative treatments. It could encourage them to approach such treatments not solely with skepticism but with an investigative openness—leading to potential innovations in integrative medicine.

In the end, synthesizing research and anecdotes doesn't merely compile information; it narrates a more comprehensive and human story. A story that might illustrate how differing strands of evidence—clinical trials and personal experiences—widen our understanding of health and healing, urging us to honor what each can uniquely contribute.

As we proceed to build upon the foundation laid in this synthesis, we'll continue to keep both empirical and personal elements in sight, aware that each step forward in this discourse contributes a vital piece to the mosaic of medical understanding and patient care.

Together, they fortify a narrative not grounded in certainty but anchored in pursuit, reflection, and an unwavering commitment to holistic truth.

Building a Comprehensive Case

In the realm of alternative medicine, compiling evidence often feels like assembling a complex puzzle where each piece represents a study, a personal account, or a historical precedent. To construct a comprehensive case, one must delve deep into various sources, from scientific journals to patient testimonials, ensuring a holistic perspective that bridges conventional wisdom with novel hypotheses.

When we consider the compelling narrative behind treatments like the synergy of gold and selenium, the first step in building a case is a thorough exploration of available scientific literature. This involves scrutinizing peer-reviewed studies that discuss the biochemical interactions of these elements, their medical implications, and their potential as therapeutic agents. Scientific journals are a trove of information, providing quantitative data and detailed insights that form the bedrock of any robust argument. However, these studies must be interpreted with caution, understanding their limitations and potential biases.

Historically, the medicinal use of gold and selenium isn't a novel concept. Ancient civilizations, from the Egyptians to the Chinese, documented the usage of gold in various forms as a therapeutic agent. This historical context adds a layer of depth and intrigue to modern studies, suggesting potential avenues for research that blend ancient knowledge with contemporary science. Furthermore, recounting these historical uses highlights the enduring fascination humans have had with these elements long before modern medicine took shape.

Yet, the tapestry of evidence is incomplete without anecdotal inputs from patients and healthcare professionals who have ventured beyond conventional treatments. Their stories often provide insights that clinical trials cannot capture. These narratives are sometimes dismissed in scientific circles as they lack methodological rigor. However, their value lies in highlighting real-world applications and outcomes that inspire further investigation or hypotheses.

To approach this task, it's vital to apply rigorous scientific methodologies. This means not just accepting anecdotal evidence and historical texts at face value but questioning them rigorously and placing them in the context of modern science. Building a comprehensive case requires one to adopt a mindset that balances skepticism with open-mindedness, ensuring that each piece of information is considered yet critically analyzed. This approach mirrors the investigative style employed in journalism, where the truth lies in the synthesis of observed facts and unwavering scrutiny.

In bridging different worlds of knowledge—scientific and traditional—one is often confronted with controversies and criticisms. The skepticism surrounding alternative treatments can stem from their historical associations with pseudoscience or due to the bleak outcomes of improperly conducted studies. Addressing these criticisms requires transparency in methodology and an adherence to scientific rigor, which ultimately strengthens the case by eliminating doubts about the validity of the conclusions drawn.

Additionally, a comprehensive case should also consider the regulatory aspects and ethical dilemmas surrounding alternative treatments. Legal cases and precedents provide context about the acceptability and boundaries of using such treatments within the conventional medical framework. Exploring these aspects ensures that while building a case, one doesn't deviate from ethical considerations that govern medical practices.

It's not only the amalgamation of facts and figures that fortifies the case but also the way these are communicated. Crafting a narrative that captures the complexity and nuance of research while remaining accessible and informative is essential. This involves presenting the case in a manner that is engaging, bridging the gap between dense scientific discourse and public understanding.

In conclusion, building a comprehensive case for treatments involving gold and selenium demands a multifaceted approach, intertwining historical insights, modern scientific research, and real-world experiences. It advocates for a harmonious integration of knowledge across domains, ensuring a balanced and informed perspective that doesn't just inform but also challenges existing beliefs. Only with such a well-rounded foundation can we hope to influence perceptions and inspire both acceptance and further inquiry into the potential of these fascinating elements in the world of medicine.

Conclusion

As we conclude this exploration into the realms of health intertwined with the mystical elements of gold and selenium, we've traversed a landscape rich with history, controversy, and scientific inquiry. The journey has not only been one of learning but also of questioning conventional wisdom, the status quo, and the boundaries of what modern medicine considers possible. We've delved into a fascinating amalgamation of ancient alchemical practices and cutting-edge scientific research, uncovering the nuanced complexities that these elements offer in the realm of alternative medicine.

One of the overarching themes that emerged throughout this discourse is the intricate relationship between historical beliefs and contemporary science. Gold and selenium, revered in centuries past for their mystical and curative properties, are again at the forefront of health innovation. Yet, the progress from enigmatic substances to potential therapeutic agents has not been linear, nor without its critics. The ties that bind modern-day health protocols with ancient remedies are as variable as the individuals who choose to explore them.

Our exploration has also highlighted the pivotal role of skepticism in scientific advancement. The medical community, while often cautious, benefits from challenging established norms. This skepticism drives the need for robust clinical trials, peer reviews, and ethical considerations. Without such rigorous scrutiny, the risk of misinformation and false hope proliferates. Yet, in a landscape that craves quick solutions, the allure of gold and selenium as miraculous cures can't be dismissed outright, warranting a balanced, informed discussion.

Furthermore, the integration of alternative and traditional medicine poses both opportunities and challenges. The blending of these worlds can enhance patient outcomes, offering holistic care strategies that treat beyond just the symptoms. However, finding that balance requires careful navigation through regulatory, ethical, and cultural landscapes. The stories of recovery and patient testimonies provide powerful narratives, yet they must be tempered with scientific evidence and standard medical advice.

The potential synergistic effects of gold and selenium, as discussed, invite further research and optimism. While the biochemistry behind their interactions remains complex, preliminary studies suggest a realm of possibilities. These elements might offer adjunctive options, especially in cancer treatment and prevention, providing hope where conventional treatments fall short. Yet, such potential must be weighed against the risks and side effects that accompany any potent treatment.

Education and awareness emerge as crucial components in fostering a well-informed public. Health policy, community impacts, and advocacy strategies play significant roles in guiding perceptions and implementation of alternative therapies. Building public understanding based on evidence rather than myth is essential for gaining acceptance and ensuring safe application.

Looking to the future, technological advancements will undeniably play a key role in unlocking further insights into the utility of alternative treatments like gold and selenium. Innovations in research methods promise to refine our understanding, potentially bringing these elements closer to mainstream medical practice. This future is not just a question of scientific progress but also of ethical stewardship and responsible advocacy.

Ultimately, as we synthesize the findings, case studies, and personal anecdotes documented throughout this book, a comprehensive narrative unfolds. It's a narrative that emphasizes the importance of open-minded investigation while remaining rooted in scientific methodology and critical thinking. The journey of gold and selenium in medicine, from ancient fascination to modern inquiry, shines a light on the broader quest to enhance human health through curious and adaptive means.

Appendix A: Appendix

In this appendix, we've compiled a thoughtfully curated list of resources that can serve as a guide for those looking to delve deeper into the intricate relationship between gold, selenium, and their roles in both traditional and alternative medicine. While the main chapters provide a comprehensive overview of these topics, this section offers an extended pathway for exploration, allowing readers to access academic journals, respected books, and credible online sources that underpin this book's findings. By directing attention to these supplemental materials, deeply rooted in ongoing scientific inquiry and historical context, we aim to empower readers, whether they're health-conscious individuals or practitioners in the medical field, with the tools necessary to further investigate and question the potential of these elements in modern healthcare. Always consider these resources as a bridge—linking the factual and anecdotal evidence discussed within the book to broader, often multifaceted, worlds of alternative treatment approaches.

Resources for Further Reading

In the labyrinthine journey of exploring alternative medicine, as presented in the main section of this appendix, it's crucial to dig deeper into the discourse by engaging with resources that can widen our perspectives. This curated list of further readings is crafted to offer nuanced insights into subjects like monoatomic gold, selenium, and their expansive roles, as well as the overarching themes of alternative medicine's integration with conventional practices. While the text you've just traversed allows a foundational understanding, these resources will plunge you into depths the book could only hint at, unlocking new pathways of knowledge and inquiry.

Begin with seminal texts and journals that engage with the scientific and historical contexts of monoatomic elements. One such publication is the "Journal of Medicinal Chemistry," which often includes rigorous studies on gold compounds and their biochemical properties. Here, researchers explore not just the chemistry, but the profound implications these elements have in medicinal applications. These articles provide a springboard into the potential and verified capabilities of gold in a medical setting, bridging ancient beliefs with contemporary science.

For historical perspectives on gold used as medicine, consider delving into "Alchemy and the Medicine of Antiquity" by Dr. Carla De Giovanni, a historian who intricately details the alchemical practices across civilizations and their transformative impacts on medical practices. It's a compelling read that embeds alchemy within a broader historical framework, offering insights into how alchemical processes were perceived and utilized.

Selenium's role in health and medicine finds substantial coverage in the "American Journal of Clinical Nutrition." This journal frequently publishes studies unraveling selenium as an essential nutrient and its acclaimed miracle-like properties in fighting cancer and other ailments. For those intrigued by selenium's narrative in modern medicine, these papers are indispensable in understanding its biochemical significance alongside real-world clinical applications.

Explore "The Science of Early Alchemical Practices" by Thomas H. Wright for a thorough analysis of how ancient alchemical practices are being rediscovered and repurposed in contemporary therapeutic settings. Wright's work is both scholarly and approachable, shedding light on the mystical practices of old and their surprising validation in modern labs. His chapters on translating ancient methods to modern medicine could be particularly enlightening.

Oncology researchers and clinicians interested in the intersection of gold and cancer treatment should consider "Gold-Based Therapeutics: Future Directions and Applications," a comprehensive review delving into recent clinical studies and trials. This book provides a platform to critically assess the therapeutic potential and limitations of gold compounds in cancer treatment, offering extensive bibliographies and case studies that can be gold mines of information.

The controversy and skepticism surrounding alternative treatments are being navigated expertly in books such as "Alternative Medicine: Critical Reflections and Ethical Perspectives" by Sarah L. Jenkins. Jenkins' work addresses the ethical dilemmas and controversies often surrounding alternative treatments, advocating for a balanced view that champions both scientific rigor and patient autonomy.

To gather extensive information on how modern science regards alternative medicine, "Evidence-Based Approaches to Alternative Therapies" is a must-read. This volume offers a comprehensive look at clinical trials, adding layers of understanding on the methodologies employed to test the efficacy and safety of unconventional treatments. It's a critical resource for anyone interested in peer-reviewed outcomes and statistical analyses that support or debunk alternative medical claims.

For those with an interest more finely attuned to the regulation and legal aspects of using alternative treatments, "Medical Law and Ethics in Alternative Medicine" explores legal cases and regulatory challenges physicians and patients face globally. It's an essential resource to understand the complexities of navigating healthcare systems when it comes to integrative medicine.

Lastly, the psychological and mental health dimensions of healing with alternative medicine forms an important area of study. "Mind-Body Medicine: Foundations and Evidence," written by esteemed psychologist Dr. Helen Marcus, provides a scientific backing to the psychological benefits often reported by patients undergoing alternative therapies. Her work synthesizes an array of studies, offering an empirical basis to often anecdotal claims.

Armed with these resources, the curious can delve further into the multi-faceted world of monoatomic elements, selenium, and alternative medicine. As this journey evolves, these readings not only augment the foundational understanding laid out in this book but also challenge you to continually question, explore, and expand your horizons in the intricate tapestry of alternative and integrative medicine.

Glossary of Terms

- **Alchemy:** A philosophical tradition the root of which lies in transforming matter. Historically associated with efforts to turn base metals into gold and achieving healing and spiritual enlightenment.

- **Alternative Medicine:** Practices in healing that fall outside conventional western medical methods. These can include herbal remedies, acupuncture, and other non-traditional methods.

- **Biochemical Interactions:** Chemical processes occurring within living organisms that affect bodily functions. In this context, it refers to how elements like gold and selenium might work at a molecular level.

- **Clinical Trials:** Research studies conducted with human volunteers aimed at evaluating a medical, surgical, or behavioral intervention. Essential for determining the efficacy of new treatments.

- **Holistic Approaches:** Healthcare practices that emphasize the connection of mind, body, and spirit while treating the whole person, not just symptoms and disease.

- **Monoatomic Gold:** A form of gold consisting of single atoms not bound to each other, allegedly having unique properties and uses in health treatments.

- **Nutritional Supplementation:** The process of taking vitamins, minerals, herbs, or other substances to enhance one's diet and promote health.

- **Peer Review:** The evaluation of work by one or more people with similar competencies, serving as a form of self-regulation and quality control in scientific research.

- **Selenium:** A trace mineral essential for human health, playing a critical role in metabolism and serving as an antioxidant.

- **Synergistic Effects:** When two substances interact to produce a combined effect greater than the sum of their separate effects.

- **The Mind-Body Connection:** The thought that the state of the mind can affect the state of the body, playing a significant role in health and illness.

This glossary provides clarity on terms central to understanding the intersections of traditional medicine, alternative therapies, and the specific roles that elements like gold and selenium play in modern health conversations.

Clinical Trial Summaries

In the realm of alternative medicine and integrated health, the scrutiny of clinical trials becomes crucial. These trials form the backbone of evidence-based approaches, lending credibility and providing insights into the safety and efficacy of treatments. *Clinical trial summaries* for enhanced familiarity guide the reader through complex scientific information. They do so by distilling details into clear, concise explanations.

Clinical trials can be classified into several phases, each designed to answer specific questions while evaluating a treatment's overall potential. Phase I trials are primarily concerned with assessing safety. Here, the emphasis is on defining the safest dosage range and identifying potential side effects. The small sample size allows for close monitoring of participants. Phase II transitions focus slightly towards efficacy while continuing safety evaluations.

When moving on to Phase III trials, the stakes elevate. Researchers must compare new treatments against the current standard of care in a much larger cohort. The diversity in participants helps in determining if the treatment works universally or only in specific subgroups. Finally, Phase IV trials occur after a treatment gets approval for public use. These studies continue to monitor the long-term effects and benefits, ensuring that the treatment remains safe over time.

The nuances of alternative treatments like monoatomic gold and selenium highlight how trials must adapt to the unique qualities of each compound. With monoatomic gold, for instance, trials examine bioavailability, the body's ability to absorb and utilize the element, and potential metabolic effects. Such trials might span weeks or even months, scrutinizing changes in participant health markers.

In selenium trials, researchers explore its antioxidant properties and its potential role in preventing cancer. Here, dosages vary widely depending on the individual's existing nutrient levels and health status. Some trials investigate the potential synergistic effects when selenium is combined with other nutrients or treatments. This demands rigorous patient selection and tailored protocols.

The methodologies at play in these trials often involve a controlled environment, where variables are meticulously managed. Randomized, double-blind, placebo-controlled trials are the gold standard, ensuring that neither participants nor researchers are biased in their observations or interpretations. These conditions help validate results, making them more widely acceptable within the scientific community.

Yet, the path from trial conception to publication is rarely straightforward. Ethical considerations must be handled with care, especially in trials involving patients with serious health conditions. Informed consent becomes a critical step, ensuring participants understand the potential risks and benefits of participating in the study.

Moreover, trials are often subject to peer review—a rigorous process that seeks to verify the accuracy and reliability of findings before they are published in medical journals. Only studies that withstand the scrutiny of the broader scientific community move forward in influencing clinical practice.

While many trials conclude with clear results, others might yield more questions than answers. In such cases, follow-up studies may delve deeper into unresolved issues, refine dosage recommendations, or explore combination therapies that could enhance treatment effectiveness. As researchers share their findings, ongoing dialogue within the medical community fosters further investigation, leading to new trials and continuous improvement in care.

The outcomes from these trials eventually contribute to treatment guidelines that medical professionals rely on. However, it is essential to remember that clinical trials are inherently human endeavors, subject to limitations and sometimes unexpected outcomes. They reflect the complexity of biological systems and the challenges of translating scientific discovery into healing.

In exploring the clinical trial summaries for monoatomic gold and selenium, this book aims to offer not just an understanding of the data but a narrative that ties together the journey of these elements from under-researched alternatives to their current standing in the medical field. As more research emerges, these summaries may one day reflect the significant impact these elements have made on modern health paradigms.

Ultimately, the summaries serve as a testament to the perseverance of medical innovation, driven by curiosity and a relentless quest for knowledge. They illuminate how each trial, in its detailed inquiry and patient-centered approach, adds a new layer of understanding, paving the way for future breakthroughs in both alternative and conventional medicine.

THE 15 PRAYERS OF ST. BRIDGET

These Prayers and these Promises have been copied from a book printed in Toulouse in 1740 and published by the P. Adrien Parvilliers of the Company of Jesus, Apostolic Missionary of the Holy Land, with approbation, permission and recommendation to distribute them.
Pope Pius IX took cognisance of these Prayers with the prologue; he approved them May 31, 1862, recognising them as true and for the good of souls.

As St. Bridget for a long time wanted to know the number of blows Our Lord received during His Passion, He one day appeared to her and said: "I received 5480 blows on My Body. If you wish to honour them in some way, say 15 Our Fathers and 15 Hail Marys with the following Prayers (which He taught her) for a whole year. When the year is up, you will have honoured each one of My Wounds."

He made the following promises to anyone who recited these Prayers for a whole year:

1. I will deliver 15 souls of his lineage from Purgatory.
2. 15 souls of his lineage will be confirmed and preserved in grace.
3. 15 sinners of his lineage will be converted.
4. Whoever recites these Prayers will attain the first degree of perfection.
5. 15 days before his death I will give him My Precious Body in order that he may escape eternal starvation; I will give him My Precious Blood to drink lest he thirst eternally.
6. 15 days before his death he will feel a deep contrition for all his sins and will have a perfect knowledge of them.
7. I will place before him the sign of My Victorious Cross for his help and defence against the attacks of his enemies.
8. Before his death I shall come with My Dearest Beloved Mother.
9. I shall graciously receive his soul, and will lead it into eternal joys.
10. And having led it there I shall give him a special draught from the fountain of My Deity, something I will not for those who have not recited My Prayers.
11. Let it be known that whoever may have been living in a state of mortal sin for 30 years, but who will

recite devoutly, or have the intention to recite these Prayers, the Lord will forgive him all his sins.

12. I shall protect him from strong temptations.
13. I shall preserve and guard his 5 senses.
14. I shall preserve him from a sudden death.
15. His soul will be delivered from eternal death.
16. He will obtain all he asks for from God and the Blessed Virgin.
17. If he has lived all his life doing his own will and he is to die the next day, his life will be prolonged.
18. Every time one recites these Prayers he gains 100 days indulgence.
19. He is assured of being joined to the supreme Choir of Angels.
20. Whoever teaches these Prayers to another, will have continuous joy and merit which will endure eternally.
21. There where these Prayers are being said or will be said in the future God is present with His grace.

Each prayer is preceded by one Our Father and one Hail Mary.

Our Father, who art in heaven, hallowed be thy name.
Thy kingdom come.
Thy will be done on earth as it is in heaven.
Give us this day our daily bread and forgive us our trespasses as we forgive those who trespass against us and lead us not into temptation but deliver us from evil. **Amen**

Hail Mary, full of grace, the Lord is with thee; blessed art thou among women and blessed is the fruit of thy womb, Jesus.
Holy Mary, Mother of God, pray for us sinners, now and at the hour of our death. **Amen.**

FIRST PRAYER

Our Father - Hail Mary.
O Jesus Christ! Eternal Sweetness to those who love Thee,
joy surpassing all joy and all desire, Salvation and Hope of
all sinners, Who hast proved that Thou hast no greater
desire than to be among men, even assuming human nature
at the fullness of time for the love of men, recall all the
sufferings Thou hast endured from the instant of Thy
conception, and especially during Thy Passion, as it was
decreed and ordained from all eternity in the Divine plan.

Remember, O Lord, that during the Last Supper with Thy
disciples, having washed their feet, Thou gavest them Thy
Most Precious Body and Blood, and while at the same time
thou didst sweetly console them, Thou didst foretell them
Thy coming Passion.
Remember the sadness and bitterness which Thou didst
experience in Thy Soul as Thou Thyself bore witness saying:
"My Soul is sorrowful even unto death."

Remember all the fear, anguish and pain that Thou didst
suffer in Thy delicate Body before the torment of the
Crucifixion, when, after having prayed three times, bathed
in a sweat of blood, Thou wast betrayed by Judas, Thy
disciple, arrested by the people of a nation Thou hadst
chosen and elevated, accused by false witnesses, unjustly
judged by three judges during the flower of Thy youth and
during the solemn Paschal season.

Remember that Thou wast despoiled of Thy garments and
clothed in those of derision; that Thy Face and Eyes were
veiled, that Thou wast buffeted, crowned with thorns, a reed
placed in Thy Hands, that Thou was crushed with blows and
overwhelmed with affronts and outrages.
In memory of all these pains and sufferings which Thou didst
endure before Thy Passion on the Cross, grant me before my
death true contrition, a sincere and entire confession,
worthy satisfaction and the remission of all my sins. **Amen.**

SECOND PRAYER
Our Father – Hail Mary.
O Jesus! True liberty of angels, Paradise of delights, remember the horror and sadness which Thou didst endure when Thy enemies, like furious lions, surrounded Thee, and by thousands of insults, spits, blows, lacerations and other unheard-of-cruelties, tormented Thee at will.

In consideration of these torments and insulting words, I beseech Thee, O my Saviour, to deliver me from all my enemies, visible and invisible, and to bring me, under Thy protection, to the perfection of eternal salvation. **Amen.**

THIRD PRAYER
Our Father – Hail Mary.
O Jesus! Creator of Heaven and earth Whom nothing can encompass or limit, Thou Who dost enfold and hold all under Thy Loving power, remember the very bitter pain.

Thou didst suffer when the Jews nailed Thy Sacred Hands and Feet to the Cross by blow after blow with big blunt nails, and not finding Thee in a pitiable enough state to satisfy their rage, they enlarged Thy Wounds, and added pain to pain, and with indescribable cruelty stretched Thy Body on the Cross, pulled Thee from all sides, thus dislocating Thy Limbs.

I beg of Thee, O Jesus, by the memory of this most Loving suffering of the Cross, to grant me the grace to fear Thee and to Love Thee. **Amen.**

FOURTH PRAYER
Our Father – Hail Mary.
O Jesus! Heavenly Physician, raised aloft on the Cross to heal our wounds with Thine, remember the bruises which

Thou didst suffer and the weakness of all Thy Members which were distended to such a degree that never was there pain like unto Thine.

From the crown of Thy Head to the Soles of Thy Feet there was not one spot on Thy Body that was not in torment, and yet, forgetting all Thy sufferings, Thou didst not cease to pray to Thy Heavenly Father for Thy enemies, saying: "Father forgive them for they know not what they do."

Through this great Mercy, and in memory of this suffering, grant that the remembrance of Thy Most Bitter Passion may effect in us a perfect contrition and the remission of all our sins. **Amen**.

FIFTH PRAYER
Our Father – Hail Mary.
O Jesus! Mirror of eternal splendour, remember the sadness which Thou experienced, when contemplating in the light of Thy Divinity the predestination of those who would be saved by the merits of Thy Sacred Passion.

Thou didst see at the same time, the great multitude of reprobates who would be damned for their sins, and Thou · didst complain bitterly of those hopeless lost and unfortunate sinners.

Through this abyss of compassion and pity, and especially through the goodness which Thou displayed to the good thief when Thou saidst to him: "This day, thou shalt be with Me in Paradise." I beg of Thee, O Sweet Jesus, that at the hour of my death, Thou wilt show me mercy. **Amen**.

SIXTH PRAYER
Our Father – Hail Mary.
O Jesus! Beloved and most desirable King, remember the

grief Thou didst suffer, when naked and like a common criminal.

Thou was fastened and raised on the Cross, when all Thy relatives and friends abandoned Thee, except Thy Beloved Mother, who remained close to Thee during Thy agony and whom Thou didst entrust to Thy faithful disciple when Thou saidst to Mary: "Woman, behold thy son!" and to St. John: "Son, behold thy Mother!"

I beg of Thee O my Saviour, by the sword of sorrow which pierced the soul of Thy holy Mother, to have compassion on me in all my affliction and tribulations, both corporal and spiritual, and to assist me in all my trials, and especially at the hour of my death. **Amen**.

SEVENTH PRAYER
Our Father – Hail Mary.
O Jesus! Inexhaustible Fountain of compassion, Who by a profound gesture of Love, said from the Cross: "I thirst!" suffered from the thirst for the salvation of the human race.

I beg of Thee O my Saviour, to inflame in our hearts the desire to tend toward perfection in all our acts; and to extinguish in us the concupiscence of the flesh and the ardor of worldly desires. **Amen**.

EIGHTH PRAYER
Our Father – Hail Mary.
O Jesus! Sweetness of hearts, delight of the spirit, by the bitterness of the vinegar and gall which Thou didst taste on the Cross for Love of us, grant us the grace to receive worthily.

Thy Precious Body and Blood during our life and at the hour of our death, that they may serve as a remedy and consolation for our souls. **Amen.**

NINTH PRAYER
Our Father – Hail Mary.
O Jesus! Royal virtue, joy of the mind, recall the pain Thou didst endure when, plunged in an ocean of bitterness at the approach of death, insulted, outraged by the Jews.

Thou didst cry out in a loud voice that Thou was abandoned by Thy Father, saying: "My God, My God, why hast Thou forsaken me?"

Through this anguish, I beg of Thee, O my Saviour, not to abandon me in the terrors and pains of my death. **Amen.**

TENTH PRAYER
Our Father – Hail Mary.
O Jesus! Who art the beginning and end of all things, life and virtue, remembers that for our sakes Thou was plunged in an abyss of suffering from the soles of Thy Feet to the crown of Thy Head.

In consideration of the enormity of Thy Wounds, teach me to keep, through pure love, Thy Commandments, whose way is wide and easy for those who love Thee. **Amen.**

ELEVENTH PRAYER
Our Father – Hail Mary.
O Jesus! Deep abyss of mercy, I beg of Thee, in memory of Thy Wounds which penetrated to the very marrow of Thy Bones and to the depth of Thy being, to draw me, a miserable sinner, overwhelmed by my offenses, away from sin and to hide me from Thy Face justly irritated against me, hide me in Thy wounds, until Thy anger and just indignation shall have passed away. **Amen.**

TWELFTH PRAYER
Our Father – Hail Mary.
O Jesus! Mirror of Truth, symbol of unity, bond of charity, remember the multitude of wounds with which Thou wast afflicted from head to foot, torn and reddened by the spilling of Thy adorable Blood. O great and universal pain, which Thou didst suffer in Thy virginal flesh for love of us! Sweetest Jesus! What is there that Thou couldst have done for us which Thou has not done!

May the fruit of Thy suffering be renewed in my soul by the faithful remembrance of Thy Passion, and may Thy love increase in my heart each day, until I see Thee in eternity: Thou Who art the treasure of every real good and every joy, which I beg Thee to grant me, O Sweetest Jesus, in heaven. **Amen.**

THIRTEENTH PRAYER
Our Father – Hail Mary.
O Jesus! Strong Lion, Immortal and Invincible King, remember the pain which Thou didst endure when all Thy strength, both moral and physical, was entirely exhausted, Thou didst bow Thy Head, saying: "It is consummated!"

Through this anguish and grief, I beg of Thee Lord Jesus, to have mercy on me at the hour of my death when my mind will be greatly troubled and my soul will be in anguish. **Amen.**

FOURTEENTH PRAYER
Our Father – Hail Mary.
O Jesus! Only Son of the Father, Splendour and Figure of His Substance, remember the simple and humble recommendation.

Thou didst make of Thy Soul to Thy Eternal Father, saying: "Father, into Thy Hands I commend My Spirit!" And with Thy Body all torn, and Thy Heart Broken, and the bowels of Thy Mercy open to redeem us, Thou didst Expire.

By this Precious Death, I beg of Thee O King of Saints, comfort me and help me to resist the devil, the flesh and the world, so that being dead to the world I may live for Thee alone.

I beg of Thee at the hour of my death to receive me, a pilgrim and an exile returning to Thee. **Amen.**

FIFTEENTH PRAYER
Our Father - Hail Mary.
O Jesus! True and fruitful Vine! Remember the abundant outpouring of Blood which Thou didst so generously shed from Thy Sacred Body as juice from grapes in a wine press.

From Thy Side, pierced with a lance by a soldier, blood and water issued forth until there was not left in Thy Body a single drop, and finally, like a bundle of myrrh lifted to the top of the Cross Thy delicate Flesh was destroyed, the very Substance of Thy Body withered, and the Marrow of Thy Bones dried up.

Through this bitter Passion and through the outpouring of Thy Precious Blood, I beg of Thee, O Sweet Jesus, to receive my soul when I am in my death agony. **Amen.**

CONCLUSION
O Sweet Jesus! Pierce my heart so that my tears of penitence and love will be my bread day and night; may I be converted entirely to Thee, may my heart be Thy perpetual habitation, may my conversation be pleasing to Thee, and

may the end of my life be so praiseworthy that I may merit
Heaven and there with Thy saints, praise Thee
forever. **Amen.**